Other Endings

Other Endings

ORGAN TRANSPLANTATION
and the BURDENS *of* HOPE

Anita Slominska

McGill-Queen's University Press
Montreal & Kingston • London • Chicago

© McGill-Queen's University Press 2026

ISBN 978-0-2280-2719-5 (paper)
ISBN 978-0-2280-2720-1 (ePDF)
ISBN 978-0-2280-2721-8 (ePUB)

Legal deposit first quarter 2026
Bibliothèque et Archives nationales du Québec

Printed in Canada on acid-free paper that is 100% ancient forest free (100% post-consumer recycled), processed chlorine free

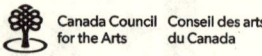

We acknowledge the support of the Canada Council for the Arts.
Nous remercions le Conseil des arts du Canada de son soutien.

McGill-Queen's University Press in Montreal is on land which long served as a site of meeting and exchange amongst Indigenous Peoples, including the Haudenosaunee and Anishinabeg nations. In Kingston it is situated on the territory of the Haudenosaunee and Anishinaabek. We acknowledge and thank the diverse Indigenous Peoples whose footsteps have marked these territories on which peoples of the world now gather.

Library and Archives Canada Cataloguing in Publication

Title: Other endings : organ transplantation and the burdens of hope / Anita Slominska.
Names: Slominska, Anita, author
Description: Includes bibliographical references and index.
Identifiers: Canadiana (print) 20250271532 | Canadiana (ebook) 20250271583 | ISBN 9780228027195 (paper) | ISBN 9780228027201 (ePDF) | ISBN 9780228027218 (ePUB)
Subjects: LCSH: Slominska, Anita. | LCSH: Liver—Transplantation—Patients—Canada—Biography. | LCSH: Sisters—Canada—Biography. | LCSH: Transplantation of organs, tissues, etc.—Canada. | LCGFT: Autobiographies.
Classification: LCC RD546.S56 2026 | DDC 362.1975/5620092—dc23

This book was designed and typeset by Sayre Street Books in Baskerville 10 Pro. Copyediting by Susan Glickman.

McGill-Queen's University Press
Suite 1720, 1010 Sherbrooke St West, Montreal, QC, H3A 2R7

Authorized safety representative in the EU: Mare Nostrum Group BV, Mauritskade 21D, 1091 GC Amsterdam, the Netherlands, gpsr@mare-nostrum.co.uk

Contents

Acknowledgments | vii
Abbreviations | ix

Introduction | 3
Learning About the Organ Shortage | 11
Do Not F--- with Me | 21
Die Waiting | 29
High Quality | 56
Death at 6:15 | 65
The Story of MELD | 78
Failure | 95
Woodlawn Cemetery | 113
The Hepatic Happening | 134
Epilogue: The Bay of Fundy | 138

Notes | 147
Index | 167

Acknowledgments

This book is based on my PhD dissertation. Thank you to everyone at Western University who supported me throughout my graduate studies, especially my supervisor, Susan Knabe, for her constant encouragement and generosity, and her trust in me to write the way I wanted to; my committee members Eunice Gorman and Sandy DeLuca; and graduate program director Sharon Sliwinski. My committee member Lindsay Bell deserves special recognition for giving me the courage and confidence to pursue this project, and for her extraordinary mentorship.

Thank you to Khadija Coxon at McGill-Queen's University Press for her wisdom and guidance. I am grateful to the anonymous peer reviewers who gave feedback on an earlier version of this manuscript that helped me revise it into a more personal story. Thank you to Susan Glickman for carefully editing the manuscript.

The love and support of my parents, Ken and Helen Saunders, has been a pillar throughout writing this book. I am grateful to my friends for believing in me. I am especially grateful to Damien Dabrowski for reading and rereading this manuscript, providing honest feedback and encouragement. I recognize my children Sasha, Neena, and Kai as the most vital elements of my life. I thank them for being who they are and for their love.

This book is dedicated to Shauna, for us.

Abbreviations

CBS   Canadian Blood Services
CPT   Child Pugh Turcotte
CST   Canadian Society of Transplantation
EBM   evidence-based medicine
ESDL end-stage liver disease
HCC   hepatocellular carcinoma
MELD Model for End-Stage Liver Disease
NOTA National Organ Transplant Act
OPTN Organ Procurement and Transplantation Network
PSC   primary sclerosing cholangitis
SBP   spontaneous bacterial peritonitis
UNOS United Network of Organ Sharing

Other Endings

Introduction

In 2003 my sister Shauna was listed for a liver transplant, the only potentially curative treatment for her end-stage liver disease. During her eighteen-month wait for the "gift of life," her health precipitously declined, and she died in an ICU. All along I had believed that she was going to receive a successful transplant and be able to start a new life. I was attuned to the stories of those fortunate recipients who were able to get a transplant and thrive, and my sister belonged to that cast of heroes and survivors.

But Shauna's death was a shocking passage to an unwanted conclusion. Redemption was out of reach for her. One friend of Shauna's sent a condolence note that read, "I simply cannot fathom that this happened"; others apologized for not knowing what to say, or opted for silver-lining messages about the richness of fond memories and relief that "suffering is over," or even fevered words about death as liberation from mortal life ("May you fly on Angel's wings!!!!!"). The condolences were sincere, but also clumsy. Everyone seemed ill-equipped to process her death.

My sister was only twenty-nine years old when she died.

The occurrence of waitlist death is acknowledged in the sense that it is tallied. Both Canada (where I live) and the US (where Shauna died) keep databases with statistics on waitlists, transplants, and "waitlist removals."[1] But statistics are not stories. The story of transplantation is focused on a transformation from sickness to health and improved quality of life. Much less attention is paid to how death, loss, and failure are also part of the story. In North America, more than one thousand patients still die every year waiting for a new liver.[2] This cumulative loss is substantial, but it largely remains unspoken and hidden.

A couple of hours before Shauna died, I posted an update in an online journal that said Shauna "had spiraled and crashed." I began the journal post almost sheepishly with the quasi-disclaimer "We don't know how to say this." I was blunt and apologetic, stating, "We had no idea that things were coming to such a bad end."

Looking back, I realize that I then viewed liver transplantation as simply being a mechanical procedure to replace a broken-down part. I also had blind faith that an act of generosity would show up eventually, get the job done, and bring a redemptive transplant story to life. The "bad end" we were faced with was dumbfounding. It felt like an erasure of everything.

"Without the organ donor there is no story" is a phrase commonly used to emphasize the value of organ donation. But the implicit message here is interesting. It's not that organ donation produces stories, but the idea that other scenarios amount to "no story." The reason I wrote this book is to challenge that narrative exclusion.

Susan Sontag writes that "to tell a story is to say: *this* is the important story."[3] The story I want to tell combines my sister's wait for a liver transplant and her death twenty years ago with my own effort to come to terms with what happened. Part of "the story behind the story" is that in 2015, I started a PhD program in an interdisciplinary health studies program to pursue research about the problem of organ donation. Shauna's death had always been the inspiration for this research, but relegating it to some unspoken backstory felt increasingly dubious. I moved towards autoethnographic writing (despite warnings from established scholars that this was "the worst thing I could do"). I made Shauna the sole focus of my study and, in the end, wrote a dissertation that was all about her.

Much of this book is based on that work.

In qualitative health research (my academic speciality), I take a "critical theory stance," which is defined broadly as paying attention to the "social, political, cultural, economic, ethnic and gender antecedents of the studied situation."[4] Theoretically, my work aligns with a critical-interpretive approach that respects individual lived experience and meaning-making while interrogating conditions that shape that experience, including the underlying structures of healthcare and societal beliefs and discourses. This approach is informed by feminist research practices that emphasize the situatedness of knowledge and knowledge production and ask critical questions about what's neglected, excluded, or devalued in the situation, and how priorities and outcomes are affected by social structures, dominant values, and power relations.[5]

In this case, it means recognizing that organ transplantation is embedded in biomedical discourse and is a value-laden sociocultural narrative, both of which condition patient and caregiver experience. I did research that supports the argument that the story of a successful transplant is framed by an ideological context that supports narratives of progress (discourses of science, technology, and medicine) and promotes the moral normativity of being hopeful. I advanced a critical perspective that the field of organ transplantation is marked by the idealization of improvement: that life can be prolonged, and death can be avoided; that science, technology, and medicine will make life better.

Avenues of critical scholarship broaden the story from being straightforward memoir focused on personal experience. Though the focus of this book is autobiographical, I have retained the descriptive context and critical analysis that shaped it and highlighted how my personal narrative has traceable threads to bigger questions and larger narratives that sometimes helped me make more sense of my experience, or validated what I was thinking and feeling, especially those aspects of the experience that seemed imperceptible or unacknowledged at the time.

A big part of this endeavour has been trying to understand why it felt so important to me to write about Shauna. Literary scholar Ann Jurecic suggests that "ordinary motives for reading and writing" are sometimes forgotten aspects of scholarship on illness writing.[6] If there is too much emphasis on how narratives are evidence of the "dominant discourse," we neglect to understand the ways that reading and writing are driven by the ordinary motives of sensemaking and forming meaningful connections. For me, much of the *important story* is beyond unpacking the social, political, and economic forces behind organ transplantation; it concerns the concrete details of individual experience and narratives of self and identity shaped by personal memories, desires, and goals.

However, I am writing from a place of knowing that no transplant story begins on a blank slate. There is no way to escape my awareness of *what could have been* but only to recognize how Shauna's experience and my experience were shaped by stories of transplantation that had already been told. A transplant story is built on a predetermined landscape that is the anticipation of a happy story. In my writing, I try to manoeuvre through that landscape and confront how after Shauna died, I felt trapped in the narrative traces of a happy story: a transplant story that was neither my sister's story nor my own.

When I started my graduate program, I wanted to address what seemed like an obvious problem: a lack of organ donations. The root issue, as I then saw it, was that not enough people donate their organs when they die. Early on, I had the opportunity to work on a project at a public relations firm that sought to better understand what messages are most effective at encouraging people to sign up for organ donation, particularly those who identify as undecided about whether they should. I conducted focus groups to elicit reactions to a variety of promotional campaigns. One of the campaigns we used in our study was "Waiting for Seven Years," created in 2013 by Ogilvy in Germany. It features a young man named Michael receiving dialysis treatment in the middle of a busy Frankfurt train station. Participants in our focus groups watched a video that documented this event as well as the media attention that followed it, namely that it brought about a 33 per cent increase in website visits and 16,000 downloads of organ donor cards and apps – a 24.8 per cent increase over the previous monthly average, according to the ad agency.

Most respondents in our study liked the concept of the ad but they also had questions about it. It wasn't the shock of this public display of hemodialysis that bothered them but the fact that the ad ended with a blank screen captioned "Michael Is Still Waiting." Some of the respondents found this to be a confusing message to end on because it made Michael's situation seem hopeless and futile. It would have been better, they thought, to end with Michael getting a transplant, to see the anticipated happy ending, rather than suggesting uncertainty about his eventual fate.

Focus groups conducted by a researcher at the University of South Carolina had similar findings. Audiences responded favourably to public service announcements in which they could "[witness] the effects of donation," namely see a transformation, especially one that included details showing that the patient was "really sick" before the transplant, such as using an oxygen tank or being confined to a wheelchair. They liked PSAs to depict first the suffering and hardship of a patient on the waitlist and then how their life was improved when they received a new organ.[7]

Without transformation to restored health, organ transplantation does not fulfill its meaning as the gift of life. Anthropologist Lesley Sharp argues that the trope of the "gift of life" is so ubiquitous and persistent that it constrains the way organ transplantation is represented and understood. While patients can genuinely feel like they want to give back by sharing their stories, this can translate into feelings of indebtedness and the conviction that they owe it to donors to share only their *happy* stories. According to Sharp, who did extensive field work among transplant recipients, patient transplant stories are "highly scripted" so that "organ transplantation is always represented as a radical and successful form of personal transformation, where the generous gifts from one person have offered renewal of life to others."[8] In our focus groups, the doubt instilled by reminding viewers that "Michael Is Still Waiting" suggested that other versions of transplantation don't belong in this narrative.

Shauna planned to share her transplant journey through an online platform called CaringBridge.org. But when she finally composed the first entry (dictated to me because she was no longer able to type on a computer), it started with the words, "Dear Friends and Family. This is not the storybook beginning to my transplant story that I hoped to write when I created the template for this page last year." She explains the "storybook beginning" would have been the call from the hospital announcing that a liver was available.

After Shauna died, I sorted through her books and found a copy of a transplant memoir that conformed to the typical redemptive narrative of suffering followed by salvation. Thumbing through that memoir, I noted that in the margins Shauna had written "trope," "trope," "trope."

Philosopher Paul Ricoeur explains that our expectations for and the imagined outcomes of any given story do not "come out of nowhere." They are handed down through tradition, and even though we could deviate from traditional models, we have a tendency of "sticking to the pole of repetition."[9] Success is the expected outcome in a transplant story because it is the product of exposure and repetition.

Shauna was in intensive care for the last two weeks of her life. The television was always on in the ICU waiting room, where I spent most of my time. One of the shows that frequently aired was *What Not to Wear*, a reality show featuring two fashion experts giving a makeover to an unstylish contestant with a wardrobe of ill-fitting, unflattering, and outdated clothes. Its basic feel-good storyline plays the same notes as the "before and after" transplant narrative. There is something bad (your clothes, your vital organ), an intervention takes place (reality TV makeover, transplant), and a joyful transformation follows (a new life with better clothes, a new life with a better organ). I can't help thinking that as I watched that show (and I did many times), I must have felt a degree of reassurance in that comforting blueprint and its resonance with the storyline I had internalized about Shauna's "second chance at life."

Historian Hayden White argues that narrative gives reality "the mask of meaning, the completeness and fullness of which we can only *imagine*, never experience." For White, "coherence, integrity, fullness, and closure" are narrative characteristics of wishes, daydreams, and reveries. They "produce an image of life that is and can only be imaginary."[10] Transplantation is not a linear story that always leads to a positive outcome. But often our knowledge and understanding of organ transplantation is limited to this "imaginary" version that posits transplantation as a rebirth. Kidney transplant recipient Rose Richards observes that "relatively little personal writing has been done on kidney failure and transplantation. A possible reason for that is that we ... are meant to fit into a happily-ever-after narrative we did not write."[11] I think this insight can explain why there is little personal writing about loss, particularly when the wait for a transplant ends with death. It doesn't fit into the anticipated narrative, and it is difficult to locate alternatives when the one "we did not write" is so dominant in the field of transplantation and indeed, everywhere else.

Learning About the Organ Shortage

When Shauna was waiting for a liver, I never thought seriously about the shortfall of organs. I was aware that the need for organs exceeded the rate of donation. Perhaps I knew that in the US, where Shauna lived at the time, eight people waiting for a liver transplant die every day. This translates into one in six dying on liver transplant waitlists every year.[1] However, this somehow didn't seem applicable to my sister. I was certain that she would be getting a liver transplant one day.

Initially, I had a hard time saying that Shauna "died"; instead, I would say that she "died waiting." This seemed like an important distinction to me. To "die waiting" implies that a transplant didn't happen in time. It implies a market disequilibrium, the supply falling short of the demand, and suggests that under better market conditions, her life could have been saved. I hoped that emphasizing that Shauna "died waiting" would make that point obvious – there aren't enough organs for everyone who needs them.

About a week before Shauna died, I called the local newspaper in Raleigh-Durham, North Carolina, where she had lived for the past five years. The helplessness of waiting produced paralysis and lethargy as well as a panicky sense of urgency that couldn't be addressed with any meaningful action. Calling the newspaper felt like doing something, a plea for acknowledgment that waiting for a liver transplant is a life-or-death crisis. That phone call resulted in a five-hundred-word article titled "To Save a Sister's Life" that was published in the *Raleigh News and Observer* on Saturday, 27 November 2004.

I don't know what good I thought would come out of this very modest publicity (a side column on the front of the B pages). The article explained Shauna was on life support, but stated that she could go back to normal life with a "new liver ... If only one would surface." I described myself as "desperate" and stated my case as follows: "What we are concerned about is this shortage and this kind of reluctance people have about donating ... We were just thinking Shauna's situation would let them know what this really means. This is not some kind of abstract notion of donating organs. This is somebody. This is a concrete person. This is my sister."

I hardly recall speaking to the journalist, though I remember calling her back shortly after the interview because I thought of something I wanted to say (I no longer remember what it was). In that brief interval, the article had already gone to press. I had grown accustomed to the attenuated pace of the hospital, so the clip of newspaper journalism was almost unfathomable to me. How could anything happen so quickly?

My fixation was that Shauna needed a donor or else she would die. It was the point of the story ("To Save a Sister's Life"). The article urges readers to donate organs and tells readers that Shauna didn't need to die; that her story "needn't end badly." The tragedy of Shauna's death would be that it was avoidable, since a cure was theoretically available. The doctors had everything within their power to save Shauna. The problem, as I saw it, had to do with inadequate organ donation.

There is no way to overestimate the monumental significance of organ donation in the lives of those who need transplants. Coming so close to it personally gave it a shadowy resonance after Shauna passed away, like I was tiptoeing around pools of darkness. I furtively signed the donor card that came with my driver's licence renewal each year. I worried that organ donation was doomed by a panoply of fears and anxieties related to mortality and the boundaries of death, as well as squeamishness about bodily integrity. I worried that most people viewed organ donation as a sacrosanct and inviolable individual choice that was none of anyone else's business. Occasionally I did little fits of late-night research on the internet. I marked my calendar for an episode of *The Fifth Estate* on CBC television called "Dead Enough" that probed into whether in all cases organ donors are clinically dead. I watched it and hated it.

I started graduate school with the objective of studying the promotion of organ donation and quickly found out that organ donation had already been overstudied, at least in certain niche areas. There is specifically an excess of research aimed at understanding what motivates people to sign donor cards and join donor registries. Coming from a humanities-oriented social science background, this type of research was unfamiliar to me. Most studies used models from behavioural psychology and tried to predict how a favourable view of organ donation can translate into signing up as a donor. For instance, a study may use the "theory of planned behaviour" to understand the pathways between "intention" (support for organ donation) and "action" (signing a donor card/registry).[2] The concept of "self-efficacy" comes up a lot. Self-efficacy means feelings of individual competency or a "sense of individual capacity," as well as the perceived ease or difficulty of completing a task. It's a perception or a belief that one is able to "enact a recommended behaviour to avoid consequences," to succeed at a task, to solve a problem, and the belief that one has the power to affect situations (whether that belief is accurate or not).[3] Supposedly self-efficacy is a great motivator – people avoid tasks when self-efficacy is low and undertake tasks when self-efficacy is high.

This kind of behavioural psychology research informs the way organizations come up with messages to promote organ donation, as well as the way they form their public campaign strategies. For example, signing a donor registry is often presented to the public as highly self-efficacious, focusing on the positive outcomes that will result from a small simple act. In Canada people register for organ donation in their provincial jurisdiction, but the national organization Canadian Blood Services (CBS) serves as an umbrella agency for organ and tissue donation and its promotion. When I started my PhD research, the CBS website homepage for organ and tissue donation addressed visitors with the question: "What Does It Take to Save Up to Eight Lives?" Underneath, the answer is simply: "Saying 'yes'" (the dying part is left out). The rest of the copy enhances the reader's perception of self-efficacy, implying that everyone who says "yes" has the capacity to save dozens of lives. It says: "Thousands of Canadians are in need of organ, tissue and eye donations. Hundreds die each year waiting for vital transplants. You can help change that by consenting to be an organ and tissue and eye donor. One donor can save up to eight lives. Tissue and eye donors can improve the lives of 75 more!"[4] Around the same time, the Trillium Gift of Life Foundation in Ontario used the slogan "It Takes Two Minutes," stressing how little time and effort organ donor registration required.

Remarkably, despite all the research aimed at understanding what compels people to sign up for organ donation, there is not much evidence that promotional campaigns for organ donation have a significant impact. Though few public awareness campaigns have been designed to allow their outcomes to be evaluated (by baseline comparison, pre/post testing, control groups, etc.) and it's hard to gauge results that aren't measurable or cannot be easily evaluated (such as exposure to the issue of organ donation), a study in the US has estimated that promotional and awareness campaigns, on average, have an overall effect of increasing organ donation registration by only 5 per cent.[5] More significantly, public awareness campaigns are almost exclusively focused on urging organ donation registration, but signing up is not the equivalent of actual organ *donation*.

When I started looking into this research topic, I had the impression that increasing organ donation was simply a matter of increasing the number of individuals who sign donor cards or join donor registries. I naively thought that when self-identified donors died, their organs would automatically be retrieved and distributed to transplant patients. However, I discovered that most people (whether they sign up or not) will never meet the medical criteria to become donors, or contribute, in practical terms, to an increase in organ donation. Only 1 to 2 per cent of people who die in hospital meet these criteria.[6] Eligible donors are quite rare, restricted to those who die in a hospital intensive care unit and are mechanically ventilated to maintain sufficient oxygen levels so that their organs are viable for transplantation.

In other words, a signed donor card does not mean you will be an eligible donor.

Historically, donor cards were intended to establish that organ donation is a voluntary and autonomous choice and thereby give individuals the right to offer their organs to others after their death as a "gift." The Uniform Anatomical Gift Act, created by US lawmakers in 1960, determined that a donor card could be used as "evidence of the gift," i.e. evidence of voluntarism (action based on non-coercion), which, along with autonomy and altruism, is one of what bioethicist Arthur Caplan calls the "ethical linchpins" of organ donation.[7] This responded to the need to garner widespread public approval for organ transplantation (back then, an unfamiliar practice) and provide a framework for organ donation that was aligned with medical, legal, and ethical standards, but it was not intended as a means to *increase* organ donation. One researcher points out that even the gift-giving analogy was never intended to be a *persuasive* message; rather "the analogy between gift-giving and organ donation was originally adopted because it was believed most accurately to capture what was thought to be the most desirable way to procure organ donation."[8]

However, being a registered donor is not akin to "saving lives," and having more registered donors does not necessarily mean that more organs will become available. In fact, a national report in Canada states: "It is difficult to link registries directly with higher donation rates." Publicity about giving the gift of life tends not to factor in the concept of "eligible donors." When I started researching this field, these facts were unknown to me. I thought the whole point of the registry was to tap into the abundance of organs from all the people who were going to die anyway. Following these revelations, I had to wrap my head around the idea that more signed donor cards will not solve the problem of the organ shortage. It was an entirely different problem than the one I had imagined.

The organ shortage was, in part, a product of the "transplant boom" of the mid-1980s. With transplant success rates improving thanks to the discovery of the immunosuppressant drug cyclosporine, the number of patients listed for a transplant began to rise during that decade, and those numbers have been rising ever since.[9] To reduce the gap between the supply and demand, it became obvious that the cooperation of hospital and medical professionals in the process of organ procurement was more crucial than focusing on the willingness of the public to be donors.[10] Towards this end, "required request" became federal law in the US in 1986, and eventually did so in Canadian jurisdictions as well.[11] This means that when a patient is brain dead, or brain death is imminent, or if a patient meets certain criteria of cardiopulmonary death, hospital staff are required to ask the family about organ donation (regardless of whether anyone has signed a donor card), making it standard practice and an operational norm. Required request has since been elaborated to include the creation of professional roles to support and facilitate organ donation in critical care units. An example of this role is a "donor physician" who specializes in donor identification and referrals and having conversations with families, and who devises and follows best practices in those areas.[12]

In the current lingo, healthcare professionals are responsible for increasing the "conversion rate" – that is, the rate at which potential donors (those who are clinically eligible) become actual donors. The problem is that the conversion rate is too low. To increase it, hospitals need better guidelines and practices to establish a "culture of donation" where all aspects of organ donation are integrated into their standard operating procedures.[13] Another strategy is increasing the eligible donor pool. The ideal donor has a fatal brain injury but is otherwise young and healthy, but these kinds of deaths are rare and so other potential donors need to be considered. This expanded pool of donors is stretched to the limits of medical viability, given factors like age and health status. The increasing demand for transplantation has led to reconsidering who is young enough and healthy enough to be an organ donor. It has also expanded eligibility beyond those who are clinically brain dead but are being kept alive by life support to include some individuals with no chance of recovery from their injuries or ailments, and who will die within a short window following the withdrawal of life support.[14]

Both Canada and the US have opt-in systems of organ donation (donor cards and registries), but functionally they operate somewhat like an opt-out system. Organ donation may be your choice, but mostly it's dictated by circumstances that are out of your control: for example, how you die, and the extent to which the hospital you end up in is proactive and encourages organ donation every single chance they get.

As a graduate student, my first foray into what I perceived as the "real world" of organ donation research was attending the annual meeting of the Canadian Society of Transplantation (CST), motivated by a "Donation Group" meeting on the program. The conference was nothing like what I anticipated. At the meeting, everyone was talking about the results of a strategic planning session that had been held the previous year regarding how to include "the voice of donation" at the CST. There were a lot of questions around "What is the purpose of the donation group?" as well as concerns about a lack of leadership, funding, and organizational support. I don't know what I was expecting, but not all this doubt and searching. There was even questioning about whether there was a need for a "Donation Group" at the CST, and whether it belonged there.

At that conference I was in the company of doctors and nurses who work on the frontlines with critical care patients and their families and assume responsibility for facilitating organ donation in hospitals around Canada. To say I felt novice and out of place is an understatement. In relation to people who actually talk to families about withdrawing life support and the opportunity for organ donation, I couldn't have felt more insignificant and unsure of my value. I met a sympathetic doctor and tried to explain why I was there. He told me that he sensed that the backstory (my sister Shauna, who died waiting), the underlying purpose of my interest in organ donation and transplantation, was very meaningful. When our conversation was over, I went to the bathroom and cried.

Truthfully, I was thoroughly disillusioned. My objective as a graduate student had been to fill a research gap related to the messaging and public education about organ donation, and I hoped that this would be regarded as socially worthwhile; however, all early signs suggested that I was probably pursuing a dead end. Perhaps, at best, registering intent to be an organ donor could make the facilitation of organ donation easier than needing to seek consent from families when the wishes of the deceased are unknown. However, research in this area had legal and bioethical orientations related to informed consent and "family override" (when families refuse donation even when the deceased is a registered donor) that were far outside my scope of expertise.[15] By contrast, as far as I could tell, there was no great interest in the promotion of organ donation registration as a research area because it was seen more as nonprofessional volunteer activity.[16] Anybody could do it.

It seemed unquestionable that I had the credibility to promote organ donation as a family caregiver with a personal story. After Shauna's death I was contacted by an organization asking about doing a piece about her, but I said I wasn't interested. I sensed they wanted a poster child, and though they were probably well-meaning, I selfishly didn't want them (or anybody) to benefit from my loss. It felt very weird and uncomfortable to contemplate that Shauna's death would be manipulated into a simplistic message about organ donation.

Do Not F--- with Me

Over the past decades, there has been little research on patient experience of end-stage liver disease (ESLD). Overall, it has been "sparingly described." Boyd et al. note this lacuna and write, "Given the plethora of complex physical, psychological, existential, social and family problems that are the norm in advanced liver disease it is perhaps surprising that so little attention has been paid to understanding and addressing the wider illness experience of these people and families."[1] The experience of liver failure can differ dramatically from patient to patient, owing to unique disease etiologies and illness trajectories. For some it is erratic and entails rapid deterioration, rendering their outlook extremely poor.

Liver failure is the third most common cause of death in the US, but only about one-third of people with ESLD are listed for a transplant. The vast majority of people who die from liver failure are never listed to begin with. The subset of patients who qualify for a transplant undergo a process of selection requiring extensive evaluation by surgeons, hepatologists (liver specialists), psychiatrists, social workers, and nutritionists. Once accepted as candidates, patients have to deal with the physical effects of liver failure and the emotional and psychological aspects of waiting for a liver transplant at the same time.[2]

In Shauna's case, I don't recall a multidisciplinary evaluation of whether she was a suitable candidate. There was no doubt that she would be listed; it was only a question of when she would become active on the list. The trigger for Shauna's activation on the waitlist in the summer of 2003 was hypertension (an increase in pressure) in the portal vein that circulates blood through the liver. Along with this alarming symptom it was obvious she had worsening signs of liver failure: lack of appetite, cramping, abdominal distention, dizziness, and lethargy.

In late November of 2003, Shauna got an unexpected call to be a backup candidate for a liver transplant. When a deceased person is medically suitable and consenting to organ donation, two recipient patients are sometimes prepped: the primary candidate and the backup. If the primary candidate cannot proceed to transplant surgery (because something contraindicating is discovered at the last minute), there needs to be another patient in the hospital ready to go to the operating room. This is because once organs have been removed from the body of the donor they rapidly start deteriorating, so no precious time should be lost on logistics and preparations that could have been sorted out beforehand.

When Shauna called to tell me she was a backup candidate, I immediately jumped on a plane to Raleigh-Durham, North Carolina, where she had been living for the past five years. I lived in Montreal, but I wasn't going to miss her transplant surgery. I was optimistic that she would be lucky. My flight to North Carolina, via Washington, DC, left in the evening. It was a small plane that was half empty, quiet, and calm. The cabin was dim with sporadic pools of overhead lights and the muted glow of screens.

Though I couldn't see much from my vantage point, the flight attendant noticed something wrong with one of the passengers several rows ahead of me. A slumped-over man could not be roused. The flight attendant requested a doctor or nurse on the intercom and, when none came forward, resorted to enlisting the help of another passenger in lifting the man from his seat, lying him down in the aisle, and performing CPR. The flight was rerouted for an immediate emergency landing and soon the plane touched down somewhere in Pennsylvania, where an ambulance was waiting. The paramedics came on board, strapped the man to a stretcher, and removed him from the aircraft. I overheard them say that he had no pulse and wasn't breathing. It seemed like such an abrupt and astonishing way to go: dropping dead on a plane, your body stranded in Pennsylvania.

When the flight arrived in DC, I was on pins and needles. I called Shauna at once to tell her I had missed my connection. She told me that the transplant had gone ahead with the primary candidate and that she had been sent home. Despite the disappointment, I knew this was the most expected outcome, plus it strengthened my confidence that Shauna would be transplanted soon. Surely if she was already a backup candidate, it wouldn't be much longer until she was the primary.

There wasn't another flight to Raleigh-Durham until the morning, so the airline put me up in a hotel. I watched a late-night movie on TV to distract myself. The man dying on the plane was disturbing. Maybe it registered that the universe wasn't giving a very auspicious sign, possibly sending a death omen, if there are such things. But

I brushed it off. Now, in hindsight, I see his death more clearly as a clue: to die up in the air, in limbo.

Waiting for a transplant is often described as a kind of limbo in which one is caught between life and death. One researcher calls it a "time paradox" – the paradox of facing life and death at the same time, explaining that the "thanatological issues" patients face can be complicated by the feeling that one is "lucky" to be listed for a transplant in the first place.[3] Research on patients' experience of waiting tends to acknowledge this as some kind of "existential crisis," but it has never been elaborately described. One study likens it to the biblical end of the world, referring to "the people of the List" as "denizens of a strange land with dark terrain" facing "their own private *eschaton*."[4] More common than this overdramatization is the reduction of an "existential crisis" to the language of disease symptomatology. One research article calls for more ESLD research aimed at "[assisting] people in an existential crisis."[5]

The remedy for an existential crisis is not obvious. One web article on a site called "Medical News Today" offers four tips for coping with or "overcoming" one: keep a gratitude journal, do not give in to pessimism, look for smaller answers, and talk it out.[6] The first two tips suggest that the goal is to banish negativity. The idea that it's bad for one's mental health to have a "negative outlook," or even ask questions that are "too big," reflects our cultural preference for optimism. This, in itself, can create the context for an existential crisis if we are continually told to "keep smiling" and "be positive" when we are faced with many good reasons not to.

Barbara Ehrenreich has offered this critique of breast cancer culture, arguing that those who feel alienated by the imperative to be optimistic and upbeat are shunned for their negative emotions like anger, despair, and hopelessness. Ehrenreich calls it the "tyranny of cheerfulness." The public face of breast cancer is dominated by hope and life (think "survivor parades") while women facing death are relegated to the shadows.[7] The documentary film *Pink Ribbons, Inc.* interviews a woman with stage 4 breast cancer who explains that celebrating those who "beat cancer" is also "painful messaging" for those facing inevitable mortality. She suggests that there needs to be more of a balance between hope and "understanding that it may not work out."[8]

Limbo is the condition of being suspended between hope and understanding that it may not work out. Ultimately, it is a state of powerlessness. Transplant patients are advised to be organized and to get ready for their transplant, but this preparation is very superficial and doesn't hold a candle to the crushing inner experience of knowing that you have no control over what is going to happen to you. Depression and anxiety are acknowledged symptoms of waiting for a transplant. But there is no treatment for the overwhelming uncertainty and insecurity involved, especially because having a precarious status related to mortality and the possibility of being saved is seen as preferable to knowing, without a doubt, that you are going to die. Unlike a typical dying patient for whom mortality can be acknowledged and accepted, the liver transplant patient is faced with a mortality that is profoundly uncertain. This can give rise to a range of conflicting emotions: anger, guilt, frustration, acceptance, denial, hope, and despair.[9]

In the months that followed Shauna's call to be a backup candidate, her condition appeared to stabilize. She became less medically urgent, and though she was still on the waitlist, a transplant felt further away. Regular life activities continued in the context of "waiting," an oppressive and consuming state that Shauna referred to in her journal as this "greedy spell of waiting."

Meanwhile, Shauna was pursuing a PhD in economics at a top US university. Despite being encumbered by uncertainty and fatigue, she continued to work on her dissertation on the history of public funding for the arts in the United States. She was conducting an economic analysis using census data and contextualizing it with social history that examined the cultural, political, and economic ideas that shaped public goods theory and federal arts policy. She was also teaching a senior undergraduate seminar that she had developed entitled "Historical Perspectives on Women in Economics." She jotted in her journal, however, that she was miserable, "shocked" at how life was still going on around her, and if she could have stayed in bed all day, she would have.

One study of patient experience of ESLD found that patients "seemed resigned to the inevitability of their suffering" because there is little that can ease their symptoms. Shauna took medication for nausea and sleeplessness, but her extreme fatigue was insurmountable. Research indicates that patients experience fatigue and lack of energy as the most debilitating issues.[10] Depression is often linked to fatigue. People feel down because they are capable of doing so little. Lack of energy and not being able to work produce feelings of loss and frustration with the limitations imposed by illness. Wants, dreams, and desires are all put on hold.[11]

Not being "productive" can also lead to loss of self-esteem. We live in a culture that measures self-worth by high productivity. The bar is high for everyone, let alone those who are ill. Shauna felt social pressure to be hard-working and high achieving, which also became a means for her to outwardly eschew illness. She was ambitious and polished, and exhibited a self-assured demeanour, all of which minimized or concealed the appearance of illness. Decades ago, Arthur Frank, author of *The Wounded Storyteller*, argued that while individuals may not feel responsible for being ill, they still feel "responsible for how they present themselves and manifest the signs of their illness."[12] Assuming this responsibility of self-presentation is a good way to understand how Shauna navigated living with a chronic illness. Above all, I think she wanted to avoid ever coming across as conspicuously needy, wounded, or struggling. Instead, Shauna always had an aura of competence. Her pain was inscrutable.

In other words, my sister largely kept her illness to herself. While concealment may have fulfilled an inner need for privacy and self-protection, these needs were also shaped by what is socially desirable – fitting in and passing as "healthy." In her case, I think this led to a degree of isolation. Deep down, I don't think Shauna was really in denial. I have no doubt that she approached the insecurity of her health with acceptance. I think it gave her an awareness and understanding that, fundamentally, there is no lasting security in life, so she was able to face her condition in a way that was courageous and brave. Nonetheless, she worked hard at what the late anthropologist Robert Murphy calls the "social skills in sickness." "As with all other social roles," Murphy writes, "a person can succeed or fail at sickness."[13] She lived up to the social standard of someone who can still thrive while being chronically ill. However, meeting this standard became increasingly hard the sicker she became. It wasn't easy for her to turn to people and say, "I'm needy." The result was that much of the difficulty related to waiting she forced herself to face alone.

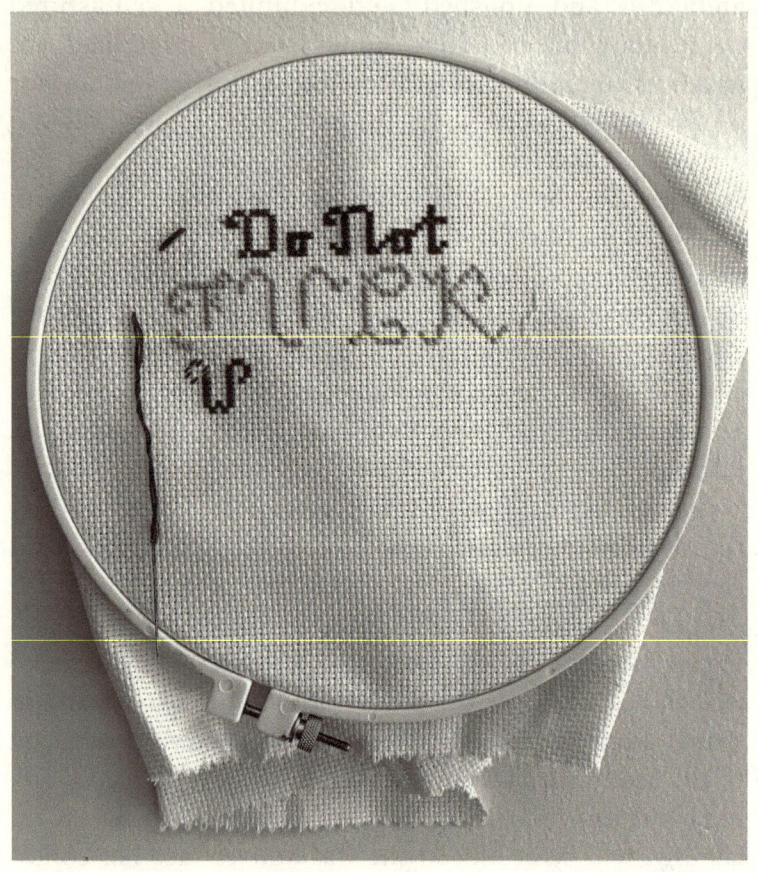

This cross-stich pattern appears to have come from a company called Subversive Cross Stitch. In addition to the lettering, the finished cross-stitch was meant to have a decorative border.

At some point, she ordered two cross-stitch patterns on the internet and started to work on one of them that says, in pastel, all caps, cross-stitch lettering, DO NOT FUCK WITH ME. The second pattern is a line of four hearts, each with a letter inside: F-U-C-K.

Die Waiting

After a year of waiting, things got worse. I didn't have a sense back then of how catastrophic ESLD could really be. My memories of that time are distorted by my assumption that things really weren't (or couldn't be) that bad. In retrospect, this has been a source of frustration. I wish I could give a more comprehensive account of Shauna's experience of waiting, but I know what I can provide is limited.

Cirrhosis impedes the circulation of blood through the liver, and this can cause ascites (the collection of fluid in the abdominal cavity). Ascites can be treated with diuretics (drugs to reduce fluid buildup in the body), but for Shauna it reached the point of being unmanageable and refractory. With the worsening ascites, her serum sodium levels also decreased: a serious condition known as hyponatremia. Low sodium causes overall weakness and has neurological impacts such as headaches and the inability to think clearly; severe effects can be seizures or coma. Shauna's sodium level dropped low enough that she needed to be treated in the hospital, which involved tinkering with different ratios of diuretics, fluid intake, and albumin infusions.

Hyponatremia also leads to complications and increased risks in surgery and post-op recovery, so Shauna was temporarily deactivated from the waitlist. She needed to meet a minimum threshold of low-normal sodium levels to be eligible for transplant surgery. In fact, Shauna's low sodium became the primary issue keeping her from transplant eligibility; it also seemed nearly impossible to correct. Unfortunately, the only treatment that kept her sodium levels from falling too low was restricting her fluid intake. Initially, her fluid restriction was manageable at one and a half litres a day, but it was eventually reduced to only 500 millilitres per twenty-four hours, about one-quarter of what an average person would drink in a day. Acute thirst became a perpetual source of torment, but Shauna endured it with stoicism because it had the purpose of getting her ready for transplant surgery. She had to pace and measure her water intake carefully, alternating taking small sips of water with moistening her mouth with a sponge. She was also offered the less dignified option of sucking on a wet rag, but I don't think she ever did this.

Very little could be done to ease Shauna's suffering overall. She regularly had a "tap," the short colloquial name for a paracentesis, to help with the discomfort of abdominal distention. This involved inserting a needle and catheter into her abdomen to drain off the excess fluid. Taps helped reduce bloating and difficulty breathing by lessening the volume of fluid in her abdomen that put pressure on her lungs. At the same time, they came with the risk of introducing infection, hitting major arteries, or piercing her massive spleen, which had become engorged with blood from the pressure on her portal vein.

Shauna's hepatologist was extremely deft at the tap and could easily remove two litres of fluid into a bottle each time he did it, but inexperienced residents were sometimes tasked with the procedure and were never quite sure of inserting the needle at the right spot. They would send Shauna for an ultrasound so that the radiologist could mark an X with a sharpie on a precise location for the puncture. While the residents approached the task tentatively, the hepatologist did it swiftly while engaged in jovial conversation with Shauna as though the procedure itself only required a fraction of his attention.

While Shauna's sodium level was stabilizing at low-normal, which permitted her reactivation on the waiting list, she caught *C. difficile*, a bacterium commonly spread through hospitals. This meant another a period of deactivation on the transplant list for the duration of antibiotic treatment. Patients cannot undergo transplant surgery with an active infection because of the post-transplant immunosuppression that is required to prevent rejection. I was now routinely gowned and gloved when I was with Shauna, as was anyone who came into her room, even momentarily. The trash can overflowed with discarded billowy and weightless yellow paper gowns.

Then came what I thought of as "another infection" – spontaneous bacterial peritonitis (SBP). This condition occurs when bacteria leak from the intestines into the abdominal cavity and infect the ascitic fluid. Whether it was downplayed by the healthcare team or just by me, it didn't register at the time that SBP is a serious complication of advanced liver failure. Instead, I was mostly bothered that Shauna was deactivated from the transplant list yet again. Following a phone call between my mother and the mother of Becky, Shauna's childhood friend who had become a doctor, my mother reported that Becky had stressed that Shauna's condition (the low sodium and the SBP) was really serious. I dismissed Becky's opinion as though she had no authority. I was in denial that major setbacks were occurring.

By that time, I had temporarily moved from Montreal to Durham. I planned to stay until Shauna recovered from her transplant surgery. I was more or less with Shauna twenty-four hours a day, trying to be useful and supportive. I kept Shauna's cramped but sunny hospital room as cheerful as possible. There were tight little flower arrangements lined up on the windowsill. I brought her duvet from home, which made the hospital bed seem a little more cozy and less institutional. She wore her own pretty nightgown instead of a hospital gown, and a lamp, also brought from home, created a more soothing ambience. These were small adjustments and transformations to make the best of the circumstances. I tried to keep all surfaces orderly and tidy because that's how she was (not me, I am hopelessly messy) and made sure she always had a hairbrush, lip balm, and other toiletries close at hand. She used an expensive hand lotion described as "an intoxicating scent of gardenias wrapped in white exotics," which, at least temporarily, gave her hospital room the ambrosial scent of an upscale boutique, masking its usual smell of drugs and the pain that lingers beneath them, bodily odours mixed with chemical agents, a combination of disease and sanitation. I lived on the chair at her bedside as constant company for her. Shauna relied on me for a semblance of liveliness when visitors came. It was my job to make conversation.

There was finally a window of no infections and sodium stable at low-normal, so Shauna was able to spend some time at home. By this point, her lethargy was extreme. She spent most of the time in bed. Her bedroom was luminous, with four large windows covered with rice paper blinds. The walls were painted a soft blue, and her bed had crisp white linens. It was immaculate, spacious and airy, like a page in a catalogue, and exuded the care and consideration she put into her surroundings. I slept on the floor of her room on an air mattress that, for the sake of tidiness, I deflated and hid under her bed as soon as I got up each morning. I was available if Shauna needed anything during the night, but she rarely did. She was still taking sleeping pills.

Shauna and I spent the time talking, sometimes listening to radio shows on NPR to follow along, or at least feign interest, in the upcoming 2004 US presidential election. We also watched movies on her DVD player. Shauna had a television on a rolling cart that was put away in a hallway closet most of the time. It came out of the closet when it was in use because she thought it was cumbersome and unsightly. We only watched what Shauna called her "encore presentations" – the same movies over and over again, mostly romantic comedies with Hugh Grant. We also binge-watched *Anne of Green Gables*. As girls, we had been obsessed with *Anne of Green Gables*. On a family trip to the Canadian Maritimes in 1985, we were thrilled to visit Prince Edward Island, the setting for *Anne of Green Gables*, which the province plays up as a major tourist attraction. We saw the *Anne of Green Gables* musical in Charlottetown and even visited "Green Gables" itself, which is to say the house in the countryside belonging to cousins of author Lucy Maud Montgomery that became the inspiration and fictional setting for the books.

I thought it would have been a challenge to find a place renting something as quintessentially Canadian as *Anne of Green Gables* in North Carolina. I opened the yellow pages with the intention of calling every video rental store in the Triangle (Raleigh-Durham-Chapel Hill) until I found it. Then the very first place I called, a five-minute drive away, told me that they had it. I was somewhat disbelieving, so

I had to double-check, "Is it the 1985 CANADIAN television movie?" Watching *Anne of Green Gables* together again reminded us that Anne, who was so earnest and melodramatic, had some of the best one-liners. They buoyed our spirits and kept us giggling.

I think back on this time fondly even though Shauna's lack of interest in watching anything she hadn't seen before surprised me, and also kind of scared me. Worse was that she could no longer play the simple word game Boggle. We tried, but it was too challenging for her, and she gave up. Shauna had developed encephalopathy, impaired mental function, because of her liver failure. In my mind, her inability to play Boggle crossed a threshold. She had reached a too-far-advanced and unacceptable level of deterioration.

I couldn't have imagined that things could, and would, get way worse.

Waiting was difficult for me but only a fraction of how difficult it was for Shauna, who was experiencing physical pain and the inability to manage it because pain medications need to be used very cautiously by people with liver failure. She also had loss of appetite, fatigue, mental impairment, gastrointestinal symptoms, and sleep disturbances. I could take daily walks around Duke University's east campus, a few short blocks from Shauna's house. This was a vague gesture at fitness and "self-care" to mitigate the growing weight of boredom, tedium, and frustration. I felt like a nervous horse circling a pen, running the fence line of a jumble of days that blended together with something like the taste of gum left in the mouth too long or coffee gone cold. On my walks, I listened to Shauna's discman. Always the same Lucinda Williams CD.

The repetition was indicative of the temporal dimensions of waiting, and the feeling that time was not advancing in any meaningful way. I think the encore presentations of Hugh Grant romantic comedies were also an expression of the constraints of waiting. Time was stuck and we weren't getting anywhere. The movies were the same and the music wasn't changing. Every time that I drove Shauna's old Honda Civic with manual transmission, *The Best of the Velvet Underground* played. Like many old cassette decks, the one in her car had "auto reverse" and switched automatically from side A to side B. This tape would soon become the soundtrack for all the time spent in a daze looking for a spot in the visitor's parking across the street from the hospital. ("It's so cold in Alaska," "It's so cold in Alaska," "It's so cold in Alaska.")

After she spent a couple of weeks waiting at home for "the call," Shauna's sodium level dropped lower than it had ever been. She was sleeping almost all the time, and in a feeble mental state when awake. Shauna was readmitted directly to the ICU. When she was feeling well enough to get out of bed, I would put her in a wheelchair and take her, and the IV tree, for a walk around the hospital. She was often cold, so I bundled her up in several layers of hospital blankets before heading down in the elevator to the atrium in the lobby for sunlight and artificial greenery. We once ran into a resident who we had seen many times during her earlier hospitalizations. He stopped for a brief chat, and I witnessed through his eyes how much Shauna's health had declined in a short time. She was speaking very slowly, a change I had already adjusted to, but it was like I was hearing it for the first time. The resident wished us well and rushed off. I continued wheeling her around the hospital, assuring myself that things weren't so bad, Shauna's strong spirit was intact. But crossing paths with that resident made me realize that I was bluffing.

I had a similar feeling of faking a sense of normalcy when I crossed paths with a hospital orderly who had once transported Shauna to radiology for an ultrasound. Shauna had been in a friendly mood with him, and they chatted all the way. When I saw him, he was pushing another patient in a hospital bed but in passing asked me, "Hey, how's your sister?" I told him she was in the ICU. He repeated incredulously, "She's in IC?" We continued on our respective paths, out of each other's trajectory, but something about his puzzlement, and the expression on his face, came washing over me: *How is this happening?* There was an unreality to how events were unfolding.

Shauna's liver was failing her completely: it was hardened, scarred, inflamed, and leaking. Her breathing was becoming more severely impacted by her water retention and she was incapable of filling her lungs to capacity. This conflicted not only with her comfort but also with her practice of mindful meditation, which was a recommended strategy for dealing with the stress of waiting for a transplant. Her workaround, she told me, was to practise her meditative breathing while pretending she was a fish, with gills not lungs, and imagining that she was doing a kind of aquatic respiration that extracted oxygen from water.

I always stayed overnight with Shauna in the hospital. Her nights were difficult and sleepless. The night shift was when I was useful by simply being there, whether we could find a silly thing to laugh about or were snapping at each other without any daytime decorum. It was unfettered and sometimes very peaceful. I could also be a bleary-eyed presence for early morning rounds, and even semi-alert if I managed to trek down to the hospital coffee shop the moment it opened, joining a long line of customers that moved according to the relaxed pace of Southern service. When I had a coffee in my hand, it felt like my first accomplishment of the day, especially if I could drink it before the doctors came.

One night Shauna and I decided to start her online journal. Over a year before, she had created a personal page on the CaringBridge website, a digital venue intended for individuals on "personal health journeys." Shauna's intention was to document and share her transplant story with family, friends, and her online support group for people like her with primary sclerosing cholangitis (PSC), an autoimmune disease that causes the hardening and scarring of the bile ducts and eventually leads to liver failure. The first journal entry is a transcription of words that she dictated to me. Shauna could no longer type, or use a pen, even with the grippy foam cylinders provided by the occupational therapist. Her once beautiful handwriting had become hopelessly shaky. Its loss was like being robbed of an intrinsic part of who she was.

The first journal entry is dated 16 November 2004 and time-stamped 3:20 a.m. It's a verbatim account of Shauna's distress in her own words:

> I would like to share with you a few things about the past few days, not sure how much I should reveal. But with that as my caveat as one of my surgical team doctors said this evening, "I am fighting for my life with my back up against the wall." I would also like to share this with you because I need your help in whatever form that might be. This past weekend in the ICU was very strange. I found myself quite unrecognizable and quite scared. Because my liver is so on the edge at the moment they have eliminated all pain killers and sleep aids that are metabolized through the liver or the kidneys and I find myself in more physical and mental

anguish than I have ever known. I continue to hold
all of my doctors in trust and realize just how much
their hands are tied as well, as they acknowledge with
all variety of bedside manner, good and bad, how they
are asking incredible, perhaps too incredible, things
from me. I trust them as they prepare for the still very
much hoped-for transplant surgery which will be a very
complicated and more risky surgery than some liver
transplants. By strange and unrecognizable I meant
both literally and figuratively. The only thing coming
through my IV aside from occasional vitamins and min-
eral supplements is saline solution and after fine tuning
different doses of diuretics I find myself with more
ascites and edema swelling than I have ever known to
the point where I have leaking sores all over my body.
The only thing that offers a blessed drop of relief is
to sit in steam and it is the only thing my doctors will
agree to. So over the weekend I was lucky enough that
ICU and this afternoon in another effort to make me
more comfortable they took me out of ICU and moved
me to the transplant wing where I would have access
to a private patient shower. My appetite is very poor
and about all that I have been able to eat is fresh water-
melon unfortunately nearing the end of its peak season
or already past. I would drink strawberry Boost if not
for the fact that that counts as part of my half litre per
24-hour fluid restriction. If anyone has any suggestions
of what I might eat at this time that would not add to
my water weight I would greatly appreciate a note in the
guestbook about these items also any tips on combat-
ting dehydration in a way that also will not add water
weight or would not need to exceed my fluid restriction,
I would love to know of these as well. Sleep as such
is not possible due to the pain and my goal instead of

sleep is relaxation and rest. Again steam helps here as well. Whatever suggestions for non-drug ways of dealing with pain would also be helpful at this time.

A few days later, I wrote: "I have been attempting over the past few days to get a chance to write another journal entry with Shauna. We have sat down together with this intent but it has been too hard – too many physical, environmental and perhaps emotional distractions. A large factor is Shauna's fatigue. Shauna misses her old self as much as we do. I think the first journal entry, which I have reread to her several times, reminds her that she hasn't lost the ability to express herself to the extent that she thinks she has." There was no time and energy for reflection, and the effort to make experience intelligible seemed impossible and overwhelming. I asked everyone to "settle for my own observations," which encapsulates the inadequacy I felt, and still feel, trying to describe what happened.

As Shauna described in her journal post, the only thing that brought her physical comfort was sitting in steam, a ritual we perfected by figuring out how to make a serviceable steam room in the patient bathroom, made possible primarily because the hospital had an unlimited supply of hot water. I also discovered an abundant towel supply in a hallway closet. I could help myself to a huge stack of towels without anybody minding (in any event, I didn't ask for permission). Hospital towels are unfortunately quite thin, so I used several layers to carpet the bathroom floor. They prevented the floor from becoming wet and slippery and blocked steam from escaping under the door. They also made the cold and sterile institutional bathroom feel surprisingly lush and cozy. Once the floor was prepped, I turned the hot water in the shower on full blast, spritzed rose water in the air, and shut the door.

While the bathroom filled up with thick steam, I got Shauna ready. I unhooked her IV, separating the line from the catheter furtively and nervously, which annoyed Shauna because she thought I made too big a deal about it. I wore latex gloves and used plenty of disinfecting alcohol wipes on all the components, but I was paranoid that I would do something wrong or kill her with an infection. I was also certain we would get in trouble, as it felt illicit and something a hospital visitor shouldn't be doing.

Once she had been freed from her IV, I helped Shauna out of bed and into the bathroom. She would sit in a motionless, drooped posture on a chair in the shower until most of the steam cleared away. I contemplated her disproportioned body and the outward signs of advanced liver failure. The upper part of her body, including her face, was becoming gaunt while her abdomen and bottom half was extremely swollen. The size of her lower legs compared to the size of her arms made her look distorted, like a badly executed oil painting. Her form, enveloped by steam, resembled a blundered work of art more than a living human creature.

I continued to communicate to a growing audience through the online journal. I reiterated the issue of pain management and sleeplessness, referred to Shauna's "strange little hallucinations" caused by the encephalopathy, and raged a bit about the doctor's concern for her nutrition. "Shauna's appetite is minimal, her mouth is completely dried out, parched, and often bleeding from weeks of thirst yet her doctors have the expectation/recommendation that she should eat like a horse to prepare herself for surgery." Shauna was so depleted and in such a dire state of weakness and exhaustion that a feeding tube was ordered. Feeding tubes are threaded through the nose, down the throat and the esophagus, and into the stomach.

Shauna, struggling to hang on to last little shreds of comfort, thought it would be beyond unbearable to have the constant sensation of a tube in her nose and throat. She refused and the doctors relented but insisted she drink the prescribed four cans of Nutrihep a day.

Nutrihep is not even food. It's "tube feed." There was something dehumanizing about having to drink *feed* (to be fair, the Nutrihep website calls it "a medical food") Whether tube feed or "medical food," Nutrihep is a thick beige liquid that smells disgusting. A friend found out that the manufacturer of Nutrihep provides "flavour packets" (banana-strawberry or citrus sunrise) but the hospital didn't have any. The doctors were okay with my DIY plan to take the cans home and figure out a way to make Nutrihep more palatable with whatever I could find in the kitchen. I simmered it on the stove with several split vanilla beans and some expensive-looking black tea that someone had given as a gift. The vanilla and the tea had strong enough flavours to mask some of the vileness of the Nutrihep. Shauna drank this concoction chilled over ice.

I knew things were going badly but I was still in denial. After all, we were waiting. Anthropologist Sharon Kaufman points out that waiting is an integral part of hospital life and it pervades patient and family experience. In the hospital, every soul is waiting for something – "for interventions, procedures, consultations, results, decisions, a change in condition." Kaufman defines waiting as "anticipation mingled with hope and dread."[1] Focusing on the hope is associated with fortitude and determination.

But it wasn't long before Shauna was back in the ICU, where the treatment goal was clearly keeping her stable until transplant surgery. This meant preventing her blood pressure from dropping while managing her difficulty breathing and poor oxygenation due to pulmonary edema and fluid in her abdomen compressing her lungs. It was a losing battle, because any additional fluid given to her in order to improve her blood pressure would escape out of her vascular system and collect in her abdomen, worsening her breathing. So Shauna was put on a ventilator. To maximize the efficiency of the ventilator, the doctors induced chemical paralysis. I explained in our online journal that "the chemical paralysis means that Shauna is not really with us. She is not responsive at all, and the machines have basically taken over all her functions. She cannot be moved, which means she has been in the same position now for quite some time, and that her gown and linens aren't able to be changed and so have become damp from her edema and ascites."

There were other problems with oxygenation and acid-base balance in her blood, and blood in her ascitic fluid, indicative of an internal bleed. Then her kidneys failed. I wrote vaguely that "there is concern right now that her kidneys have been compromised by this ordeal." The compromised kidneys were the result of a condition called hepatorenal syndrome. From the way I wrote this, it's clear that I failed to register how serious it was. Hepatorenal syndrome is an "ominous sign" that "usually portends death in days to weeks," especially if renal failure is rapidly progressing.[2] Shauna's kidneys had failed her to the point that she was put on dialysis, which I explained as a "gentle" continuous dialysis, not "full-fledged hemo-dialysis," because her blood pressure was so low. The dialysis machine was now a permanent fixture by her bed, tethered to Shauna by a thin blood-filled tube, a conspicuous stream of colour in a room with predominantly neutral tones: white, beige, grayish blue. She had to take anticoagulants for the dialysis machine to run properly, and the doctors acknowledged that this was a risky move, potentially making transplant surgery even more dangerous. The other horrid possibility, we were informed, was neurological damage, which couldn't be evaluated while Shauna was in a state of chemical paralysis and heavily sedated all the time.

The rhetoric of hope and fantasy of recovery helps manage the difficulty of dealing with the uncertainty of waiting, but it also suppresses the possibility of dying (or positions it as a "turn of events"). Hope predominated, repressing the urge to contemplate death or negative outcomes with "positive thinking." At the time, I wasn't concerned that such thinking masked a failure to accept things as they really were. I was steeped in what Arthur Frank calls the "language of survival." The imputed ending of a successful transplantation was the framework for waiting, tightly bound to a fantasy of recovery, ignoring the fact that waiting could veer into a downward spiral ending in loss.

I had generalized about liver transplantation from stories of individual good luck and happy endings, cases where the prognosis is good, so I had all the optimism in the world that this trajectory would also eventually be Shauna's. The negative outcomes weren't worth considering. There was no external impetus to question my optimism either. The imperative to be positive and hopeful runs deep in transplantation. Health researchers Sanders et al. argue that hope is more than just "positive thinking"; it is also a kind of "moral pressure" because positivity in the face of illness is a "normative moral requirement."[3]

Optimism was a mainstay of our communication with the wider social network through the online journal. The maintenance of hope often referenced God and prayers. The medical context that promotes being strong and having courage wove together seamlessly with a religious narrative that God was somehow watching over Shauna with wisdom and love. In the guestbook comments on the CaringBridge website, it was common to see well wishes phrased as "hope and prayers." We were comforted by thinking that the volume of people hoping and praying could make a difference, as though the more people were praying for you, the more likely it was that there would be "good news." At the time, it almost seemed logical. Later, reading through the abundant guestbook comments on the online journal, it seems as though we were all participants in a sham that a transplant would inevitably happen.

The bulk of CaringBridge guestbook comments and the overall mood at the time expressed an unshakeable belief in Shauna's secure future. Most people's response to her situation was to voice certainty and confidence. We acted as though we could exert control over her fate through a group investment in a happy ending, and reiterations of Shauna's strength and determination. Lumby, in her research on patient experience of waiting, found that this was, in fact, the "majority attitude." One participant in her study said, "I knew that I was going to recover, I was going to be the quickest to recover ... I had no intention of dying." Patients recall staying consistently positive, and Lumby notes that the "possibility of negative outcomes was rarely mentioned."[4]

No doctor ever discouraged optimism. This would have contradicted the central place that hope has in the cultural/moral system of dealing with human adversity. Having an optimistic outlook, as I did, seemed like an asset in the situation. In a journal entry, my father wrote: "One of the Doctors has counseled us to park our fears and anxieties at Shauna's door and carry hope into her room." According to the research, "the therapeutic value of hope is well-established." Several studies have determined that "hope helps patients emotionally endure crisis, and hopeful patients are better able to follow treatment recommendations and tolerate discomfort." However, the challenging part is to "balance supporting hope while finding ways to provide patients with comprehensible and accurate prognostic information."[5] It is not clear that such a balance is easily found, especially when "accurate prognostic information" is not what patients or families want to hear.

No one was dishonest about a transplant being Shauna's only way out, but I can't help but think that the transplant team must have known that Shauna's prospects were worse than we thought they were. Doctors tend to be very careful about what they say and measured in the way that they respond to questions, often being vague because definitive answers could be misleading or wrong. They communicated what their concerns were, but overall strived to be reassuring, while stressing caution, which was easy enough to "reframe" to "allow hope back in."[6]

Two days before my sister died, in the CaringBridge journal I was still stressing the "many reasons" to be hopeful. I wrote: "Even through our frustration and desperation we are holding on to hope and praying for Shauna. There are still many reasons to hope, not least among them that continuous monitoring has not discovered any infection. And thanks to Shauna's strength as a fighter, the surgeons still have margins to work with in her life support system and haven't maxed out." The reasons for hope were thinning: no fatal infection, margins in her life support system, and Shauna's strength/character. This journal entry represents a chain of soft-pedalled communication and wishful thinking – from the doctors to family and friends on the scene, to those we communicated with on the internet. Those "reasons to hope" now seem like a subtle form of censorship. Hope can strangle lucidity even while we insisted that it was reasonable to be optimistic. I wanted to think that I had balance and clarity, like Shauna herself, who always showed so much composure, equanimity, and moderation. But my perspective was so one-sided. In retrospect it seems fanatical.

As the end neared, I desperately clung to hope. Another journal entry says, "Shauna's Dr P came by late this afternoon. He assured us that no matter what the risks are they will proceed with the transplant when a liver is available. This is Shauna's only hope. But it is a tremendous hope, worth praying for endlessly and fervently ... We can only hope that ... Shauna is comfortable and getting ready to tap into even more reserves of strength and endurance she didn't even know she had." Shauna had become a high-risk patient for a transplant, perhaps not likely to survive surgery or recover, but this didn't seem to matter anymore. The effort to save her life was full steam ahead without much regard for the possible futility of it all.

The irrational part of the situation indicated high emotional investment and heroicized the transplant team. I regarded them as extraordinarily compassionate and caring. Trying to save Shauna's life at all costs was the crescendo of emotion and irrationality that waiting for a transplant had become. I embraced the willingness to be irrational as a form of love, determination, and betting against the odds. We say things like "I would cut off my arm for you" or "walk on burning coals" to convey passion and urgency. As I saw it, irrationality was superior because it ensconced hope. Realism made it tenuous.

The emotional intensity was blindfolding. It amplified the ending we desired (a transplant) and almost completely nullified the other possibility (dying). I also clung to a blinkered vision of post-transplant reality that made it seem like a state in which all problems go away. I don't think I registered the post-transplant reality of recovery with any depth. Though after a meeting with the transplant team, I acknowledged that it wouldn't be easy when it was presented to me bluntly. I wrote in the journal:

> Dr B. gave us reason to remain optimistic and hopeful even though we know that Shauna's battle for recovery will be extremely arduous and difficult. We all feel daunted and afraid about the post-transplant reality, particularly the knowledge that Shauna's suffering and struggling will be intensified and extended indefinitely into the future. Post-transplant, we can expect Shauna to remain on dialysis for some time, though they are hopeful her kidneys will bounce back once a well functioning liver is in place. If another system were to fail (heart, brain, lungs) this would disqualify her for transplant. Her lungs are certainly under a great deal of stress right now. A ventilator works by pushing air into the lungs, which is opposed to the way the lungs normally work, which is through muscle contraction creating a vacuum to draw in air. Ventilation certainly has detrimental effects on the lungs, and this in addition to the fluid pressure and accumulation is significantly stressing Shauna's lungs. Still, Dr B. wasn't yet worried about lung damage from the ventilator. Paralysis is helping her to conserve energy and reduces the amount of damage the ventilator does to her lungs. The other development that would disqualify Shauna for transplant is a new infection. Dr B. said that infection is his biggest fear at this time.

The risk of another SBP infection was high and required constant monitoring. There seemed to be a clear message from the doctors that barring infection, a successful transplant was possible, though I don't recall asking for a definition of "a successful transplant," or what the chances for one really were. I did reveal in the journal that "a recovery to something like a normal life is more likely the sooner a healthy organ appears, but her transplant surgery and recovery process will certainly be difficult the longer she spends on life support." I am alarmed by the vagueness of the phrase "something like a normal life" and wonder what it meant to me at the time. Perhaps I thought that everything was reversible; all the damage would be undone, and things would go back to how they were before – or become even better.

Czech playwright Vaclav Havel writes, "Hope is not prognostication." But this is definitely how I saw it. Hope represented an unambiguously positive outcome (a "new liver"), something to cling to. Havel instead argues that "hope is an orientation of the spirit, an orientation of the heart; it transcends the world that is immediately experienced and is anchored somewhere beyond its horizons."[7] In other words, hope isn't tightly bound to a specific ending and doesn't just apply to a future where good things happen. I think I have some appreciation for this definition now. But at the time, not at all.

Shauna herself had faith in God. We did not talk much about it (I am not a religious person myself) but I know she took comfort in the idea that God had a plan for her even though she didn't know what that was. She participated in an online support group for people with primary sclerosing cholangitis. It was only after we initiated the CaringBridge journal that I really became aware of how involved Shauna was in this community and the meaningful relationships she had formed there, particularly with individuals with whom she explored the topic of religion. Her health challenges had made her more religious than I realized. One support group friend posted a message reminding Shauna of a passage she had shared with her from the late Christian minister Oswald Chambers on the topic of "gracious uncertainty." He wrote: "Our natural inclination is to be so precise – trying always to forecast accurately what will happen next – that we look upon uncertainty as a bad thing. We think that we must reach some predetermined goal, but that is not the nature of the spiritual life. The nature of the spiritual life is that we are certain in our uncertainty. Consequently, we do not put down roots. Our common sense says 'Well, what if I were in that circumstance?' We cannot presume to see ourselves in any circumstance in which we have never been." For Shauna, this was a reminder not to imagine herself in scenarios yet to come but instead live with the knowledge that the future is always unknown. To fortify herself not with the anticipation of a secure future but instead with trust in God.

I didn't have this faith and equanimity. By the time the American presidential election was over and John Kerry had lost, and American Thanksgiving had come and gone, I was spending all day and night at the hospital. It was like my whole life had retracted into a bubble and the "real world" was obsolete. It was even difficult to relate to other families in the ICU waiting room. I once accepted an invitation to join some of them in an impromptu prayer circle, out of politeness I think, or a when-in-Rome attitude. I was raised Catholic, a decorous and solemn religious tradition, a far cry from this prayer circle, which was raw, almost primal, with lots of tears, trembling, and pleading to Jesus. We were all in the same boat, though, waiting for our names to be called on the intercom, the only line of communication between the waiting room and the nurses' station, letting us know that we were allowed in to see our loved ones. We wanted the best for each other, I think, but only in a superficial way. Maybe we were too submerged in our personal disasters, anxious about what news might be coming our way, frantic about who would get out of this place alive. It made us distracted, almost to the point of oblivion.

Having no energy to search for commonalities with anyone not connected to my private drama, I didn't want to be around other people. There was a conference room adjacent to the waiting room, a small windowless room with a big table surrounded by about a dozen chairs. It was used during the daytime for meetings, but we (anyone affiliated with Shauna) took it over evenings and weekends. It was also where I stayed overnight. It felt like my privileged quarters, a tiny corner in a massive institution where I had privacy and solitude. I slept on the floor in pitch blackness. I am not sure I really slept. It was something between sleep and merely lying motionless out of fear and numbness.

Technically, as a visitor, I was out of bounds, but my presence was tolerated by hospital staff. Shauna's ICU nurses knew I squatted in the conference room overnight. The doctors and residents knew too, because a team would arrive around six a.m. and flip on the fluorescent lights. Jarred awake, I would gather my things and leave them to their business. Surely it was awkward for them to encounter me there, but I felt so far out of the realm of social normalcy that it didn't faze me at all. Only once did the nurse come and get me in the night because Shauna's heart rate lowered significantly. Her blood pressure skyrocketed, quickly went into freefall, then eventually restabilized.

We used the conference room and not the waiting room as our hospital base camp whenever we could. Demarcating our own territory felt like a considerable exploit, like we had discovered a secret place to claim and to populate only with family and friends. People came.

Most of the time we did nothing. A friend taught a new (to me) version of solitaire, passed down from his grandmother, that I played frequently at that conference room table as well as in the years following Shauna's death. Even now I play solitaire to feel connected to that time. It's a small, trivial, and oddly comforting source of continuity. But it also reminds me that there was no plan, just a run of cards.

In the conference room late one night, I read the tragic obituary of Iris Chang in a copy of *The Economist* that a visiting friend had left behind. Chang was the author of a book called *The Rape of Nanking* about the mass killings and brutal torture and rape of tens of thousands of Chinese girls and women perpetrated by the Japanese during World War II. Chang was researching another book on torture, and she shot herself in the head. Lately I had read nothing, yet something drew me to read, out of all the possibilities, a piece that was harrowing, bleak, and hopeless. It must have been the depletion I felt after all the strenuous exertion to drum up optimism each day. A pendulum swing.

I had lost all contact with Shauna since she had been in the ICU. There were only two occasions that she was conscious and alert and was able to produce two shaky notes and hand them to the nurse. One asked, "new liver?" and the other note, attesting to our close bond, said, "Sister can I see her?" The latter was her last communication. From then on she was ventilated and sedated. "Sister can I see her?" were her final words.

In the ICU, Shauna was alone most of the time, in part because it was a locked ward and there were only certain times that we were allowed to see her. Each patient had their own nurse, so she was constantly monitored, but we were no longer involved in her care and had no meaningful way to intervene or make anything better for her. I wrote, "They were not letting us back to visit her very much today, as she is getting more delicate and is in need of vast amounts of medical attention. Doctors and nurses can do so much more for her than we can at this point. We are all still very hopeful that a liver is on the immediate horizon. And we are still very confident that Shauna will make it through."

Whenever family and friends were allowed in to see her, we would stand around her bed. Sitting was too awkward because at chair level you couldn't see above its sides. Standing was the only way to stare at her face and hold her small bony hand. The bed seemed very large, not like a bed at all but a commanding piece of equipment that absorbed Shauna into a nonhuman apparatus. Her body was unified with the bed and adjoined to other intensive care paraphernalia through a central line in her neck and the ventilation tube down her throat.

We were grateful that Shauna was getting what my father called the "best possible maintenance care." That phrase itself drives home that at this point she had become more like a piece of machinery. The sounds in the room were also inhuman – a hushed buzz, rhythmic beeps, and the clicking of the dialysis machine. At her bedside, I typically tried to make Shauna aware of my presence by talking to her. Admittedly, it was hard to find supportive, loving, and uplifting things to say without veering towards nervous babble, or becoming a broken record, uttering over and over again "I love you," "Stay strong," "We are here," "We are going to do this," "You are amazing ... the best ... totally awesome."

Speaking to Shauna was meant to bring her comfort because, allegedly, she could still hear us. I now wonder whether whatever awareness she had was more a source of distress than of solace. I wish I could say that I walked in there, held her hand, felt connected, and offered reassurance, but I fear my words sounded like pleas tinged with uncertainty. Once when our friend Katy and I were coming to the end of the litany of goodbyes and well wishes, Katy threw in, "Keep it real." Unintentionally, I burst into laughter. There was no "real."

Before patients are ventilated they are sedated, and their airways are numbed so that intubation is painless. After Shauna died I had a nightmare about intubation, and ever since it's been on my mind that the procedure has the potential to be traumatic. We were told on many occasions that Shauna struggled against the ventilator, which was the rationale for chemically paralyzing her. The fact that she was breathing out of sync with the ventilator and experiencing respiratory distress obviously meant that she was really suffering. Maybe she felt alone, scared, or as though she was suffocating. We constantly described her as being courageous and determined, but there is no validity to the claim that these were her actual feelings; once again, our wishful thinking was imposed on her. Once the nurse told me that "Shauna becomes agitated with any kind of stimulation." She couldn't be moved at all, which suggests that she was not in the state of peace and comfort we hoped she was but rather in a state of confusion, disorientation, and possibly fear. I minimized this because I thought that a transplant was just around the corner.

Only recently did I consider what the experience of chemical paralysis might have been like for Shauna. Neuromuscular blocking agents have the possible side effect of unpleasant awareness, so it's recommended that they are used with sedatives (to calm you) and analgesics (to kill pain).[8] I have wondered whether, under those circumstances, Shauna would have preferred to die. One night in the ICU, standing by her bed, I was overcome with a strong sensation that Shauna was trying to tell me something. I imagined that we had special powers that would allow her to say something to me through invisible channels of communication. Trying to summon this message, I "heard" her saying that she wanted to die. But, of course, I talked myself out of believing this. Ultimately, I believed that the suffering was worth it, because she was going to be saved.

After an earlier stay in the ICU Shauna wrote to friends, "I must admit that I am also very scared. I think that this past weekend I may have also experienced some of the infamous ICU psychosis or perhaps that is the same as being scared and desperate." ICU psychosis is medically defined as severe anxiety, paranoia, disorientation, and delirium. Margaret Lock explains that ICU psychosis may be the result of patients being overstimulated. She writes, "Patients suffer a complete loss of control; their bodies are penetrated in almost every available orifice and pierced in numerous places. They are subjected to a ceaseless overload of noxious stimulants, among which light and sound appear to be the most troubling."[9] At the time, I wasn't consciously considering what Shauna's experiences were really like. There was no visible evidence of Shauna's sentient self. I saw her in a nonconcrete way, like an ethereal being with a tenacious grip on the fine thread of life.

In an article in *The Atlantic*, writer Jennie Dear quotes palliative care physician James Hallenbeck, who describes death as being like a black hole. As death nears our senses fade away, but it's very hard to know the level of awareness or sensory experiences a dying person has, especially when they are sedated or comatose. Dear writes, "Being at the bedside of an unresponsive dying person can feel like trying to find out whether someone is home by looking through thick-curtained windows."[10]

In Shauna's case it wasn't just those thick curtains but also our fixation on a liver transplant that left her in a void. It was okay to me if my connection to Shauna was extinguished as long as transplant was still possible. The lack of attention I paid to her seems more callous in retrospect, given that these were, in fact, precious dying moments. My dad wrote in the journal: "We have been given another day. Shauna remains at death's door but is clinging to life on life support. The medical team feels that Shauna's life can be supported for a few more days and that a successful transplant is still possible." This message sums up how Shauna's few remaining days were measured in terms of the viability of a future transplant. This is what it means to "die waiting."

High Quality

When Shauna was waiting, we hoped for an organ offer as though somehow a disembodied liver would magically appear, surfacing out of nowhere. Unmistakably, we were waiting for a suitable donor to die. In an email Shauna sent to family and friends in the early fall of 2004, when we thought a transplant would be imminent, she acknowledged that her life now depended on someone else's death. "We humbly ask now," she writes, "that you might turn your thoughts to an unknown, grieving family that they might be guided through their time of grief and with incredible generosity, faith and love consider organ donation." The indebtedness and gratitude for organ donors is part of what makes waiting for a transplant emotionally taxing. That there are necessarily tragedies folded into the hoped-for transplant is something that I could very rarely bring myself to think about.

Once I was with Shauna for her appointment at the outpatient liver clinic at the hospital. We were waiting in the doctor's office and the door was open. One of the transplant surgeons was rushing down the hallway but stopped when she noticed Shauna, a favourite patient. After my sister introduced me, the surgeon lamented that I, so young and healthy, couldn't be a living donor for Shauna because we had incompatible blood types. "We want," she said, "to get the best possible liver for you." This was nice to hear. "Gunshot wound to the head" were her parting words. Shauna and I sort of giggled.

Of course, all transplant patients need to grapple with the idea that all deceased organ donation is the result of someone else's misfortune. But there is more to it than this. A "gunshot wound to the head" is either murder or suicide. Optimal donors are young and often die violent deaths, and there is no escaping recognizing that this is connected to a system of economic and social injustice, racism, and also mental illness. The juxtaposition of a good outcome for Shauna with a life tragically ending with a gunshot wound to the head points to a bigger, murkier picture not really being acknowledged.

Anthropologist Margaret Lock argues that the tragic deaths of organ donors are overlooked. She writes, "In North America, we proclaim a shortage of organs, even as we wring our hands at increasing suicide rates and drug overdose deaths among youth. But we do not make associations between these disparate 'facts.'"[1] In her opinion, the "gift of life" is a "seductive metaphor" precisely because it "glosses over the source of ... organs."[2] Glossing over the source of organs is also related to a wider tendency to gloss over the suffering of others. Rebecca Solnit argues that our society goes to great length to ignore it. She writes, "We come up with elaborate means of not knowing about the suffering of others and of blaming them when we do ... to be impervious to suffering you have to convince yourself that people deserve what they're getting, that their suffering has nothing to do with you."[3] While I didn't feel that others *deserved* to die, I also felt no responsibility for the circumstances that would result in someone dying in such a way that they would be an "optimal" donor. This preserved my own comfort.

The tendency to see organ transplantation exclusively as a life-saving enterprise masks the donor's death. The focus is entirely on the benefit that ensues, on "the good part" of saving lives. This blindness to loss and mortality is a form of denial and is supported by the idea that death can be imbued with more meaning if it can be endowed with life-giving legacy.[4] This "win-win" version of organ donation and transplantation has salience (and is persuasive) because it merges moral philosophy (altruism) and the rational language of economics (to maximize life-saving organ recovery).[5] It gels with our value system. Lock also underscores that the normative Western view is to see organ donation as an opportunity to "create something of value out of senseless, bad deaths."[6] With a focus on turning losses into "positive things," she argues that organ donation and transplantation represents "hopes for transcendence [and] for continuity" and can become a narrative of triumph over death for both donors and recipients.[7]

However, these "hopes for transcendence and continuity" can only be realized if donated organs are actually viable for transplantation. In reality, optimal donors are few and far between, and many organ offers are declined. One study found that 84 per cent of liver transplant candidates who die on the waitlist have one or more liver offers that are declined.[8] In Shauna's case, there were two.

The first happened the very morning she took a sharp turn for the worse. Her night on the regular hospital ward had been sleepless. Shauna, who was usually so calm, had become agitated, almost frantic, and also delirious, hallucinating we were on a boat. By morning her heart rate was irregular and she was losing consciousness. The transplant surgeon burst into Shauna's room and announced with a rush of excitement that there was a potential liver. The energy rapidly shifted when she saw the state my sister was in. She immediately ordered Shauna to the ICU and her bed was whisked out of the room so fast that there was no time to communicate with me. The situation was incoherent owing to the mix of good news (A liver! A transplant!) and bad news (Slipping into a coma?). And I just stood there, stunned, in the suddenly empty room.

The nurse gave me a large plastic bag with the inscription "PATIENT'S BELONGINGS" in conspicuous block letters and, in a daze, I stuffed everything in: tokens of comfort like aromatherapeutic room sprays, lotions, and lip balm, and small electronics like her CD player and bedside lamp. The surgeon came back to give me a hug and some kind of update that I barely grasped. I carried the bulky bag of BELONGINGS to the car. I posted a tentative update on the online journal we were keeping that stated, "events were hopefully underway," explaining that Shauna was transferred to the ICU for "surgery prep." Then we went to the ICU waiting room as we had been instructed. It was hardly how I imagined the send-off moment of Shauna's liver transplant. When the ICU team finally let us come in to see her, it was shocking. She was now intubated, with a central line in her neck, and under heavy sedation.

The transplant surgery was estimated to take place at four in the afternoon. The surgeon herself had gone to recover the liver to save time. It was in a nearby city, only one hour away. Dr W. needed to make a judgment about whether the liver could be used. It was explained to us that a "marginal liver" was being considered because, as I wrote in the online journal, "Shauna truly has no other option at this time. Since this morning she has been in a decline. She had a sudden drop in blood pressure, combined with a racing heart." I am not sure I succeeded at conveying that Shauna had plummeted into a critical state (Had she almost died?) because I used a simple dichotomy of "great" and "not great" to explain the situation. The liver was "apparently not great," Shauna was "not in great shape for surgery," but her heart, kidneys, and lungs were in "great shape" as were her strength, endurance, and fighting spirit.

We shortly found out that the potential liver had tumours, so the surgeon had to reject it. She assured us she was going to put out an "urgent call" in the region and there would be another organ offer soon. In the meantime, Shauna would be in the ICU on life support.

For six excruciating days, Shauna spiralled downward. Then late one evening, the second organ offer came. There was joy and excitement, yet we were guarded because the liver still needed to be evaluated to see if it was suitable. Also, as I wrote in the journal, "Shauna will have to survive the considerable stress of a trip downstairs for a CAT scan, which will tell us whether she might have swelling and brain damage. This would make a transplant impossible. The scan itself is a very risky proposition in the eyes of her doctors, who don't want the trauma of going through all this movement to jeopardize Shauna's stability and thus the opportunity for her transplant, but there is no other option at this point. The anesthesiologist and all of her life support – with the exception of her dialysis machine – will travel with her for the CAT scan."

Our guts were in knots. The possibility that the liver wasn't good, the spectre of brain damage, the onerous trip to radiology, how fragile she was, how easily her stability could be compromised – these were all the reasons to feel uncertain. But by midnight we had "Good news!!!" The

CAT scan showed no brain damage. I wrote, "Pray now that the liver will be okay. This is Shauna's big chance!!" The journal guestbook was flooded with supportive messages, and we were slowly elevating our hopes and expectations that the transplant was really going to happen. A couple of hours later we reported a delay due to the family gathering to pay last respects to the donor. This wasn't received as a setback. My father wrote, "We stand with grateful and humble hearts in solidarity with the Donor Family as they express their grief and say their final good bye to their loved one." We prayed for the donor family, those anonymous people determining the course of Shauna's future. The donor was already posed in the story as her saviour, bringing about Shauna's rebirth, which was now scheduled for the very next day.

We were gearing up for what some transplant recipients call their "miracle day." For my father, especially, it was imbued with religious overtones. He wrote in the online journal: "This is the day the Lord has made; we rejoice and are glad in it. Liberation from a diseased liver is dawning for Shauna. For now we wait in hope for the GO. We are excited about the new possibilities that today can bring." We waited all morning and afternoon to hear about the status of the liver. But that evening we found out it was a "fatty liver" and the surgeon was not going to use it.

Fatty liver is the colloquial name of a medical condition otherwise known as "hepatic steatosis." It sounds less like a disease than a description of a piece of meat. This was a tremendous blow, but I sent a message about the bright side too, writing, "The good thing is that she remained stable throughout the day. We also know from her CT scan yesterday that her neurological function is not impaired. Shauna is still there beneath her unconscious state. Let's hope the next offer is imminent!!! We are so hopeful that

Shauna will pull through." I also expressed gratitude, once again, to the donor family, the strangers who are part of this story.

One health policy scholar explains: "If it appears that the organ procurement agency is 'waiting for someone to die,' it's because they are. But this is quite different from wanting someone to die, and painful as the thought must be, organ transplantation depends on death."[9] That painful part is well shielded from everyone involved, largely because the practice is immersed in euphemistic language. "Availability" is a prime example of a euphemism in organ transplantation. Availability is a word that is used freely and easily. The availability of a new liver submerges the death of the donor in a feel-good narrative of survival.

In those days leading up to Shauna's death, had there been a fatal car crash or a gunshot death or a suicide, I would have been very glad because it might have meant a liver for Shauna. The doctors would have come to us with "good news." The message wouldn't be about the tragic end of someone else's life, but just about a body part that would become "Shauna's new liver" as though it had no previous owner.

In her book *Strange Harvest: Organ Transplants, Denatured Bodies, and Transformed Selves*, anthropologist Lesley Sharp describes organ procurement as a form of body commodification that transforms organs into depersonalized (and scarce) "coveted goods." She sees that transplant patients/recipients are encouraged to depersonalize organ donation and imagine waiting for a disembodied organ. Margaret Lock interprets this in terms of the Marxist notion of the fetishization of the commodity. The basis of commodity fetishism is that it renders social relations invisible. Lock explains that "the commodity – the object – is decontextualized in a capitalist system, and consumers know little or nothing about the social relations of production or of exchange." In the case of organ transplantation, human organs are "transformed into decontextualized objects. Their previous social history is erased, and their value assessed solely in terms of their quality as organs for transplant: are they vital and healthy, have they been well cared for during procurement?"[10] It's almost as though the death of the donor isn't part of organ procurement, a kind of tricky thinking that results, as Locks sees it, in the conviction that there ought to be enough organs available for everyone who needs them.[11]

Meanwhile, the family of the donor is encouraged to see organ donation as a way for their loved one to live on. Sharp frames this as an "ideological disjuncture" between donation and transplantation where competing messages and euphemistic expressions are used to describe the same processes. In her analysis, body commodification is couched in a "Gift of Life" discourse that stresses lofty values like generosity and altruism and does not acknowledge that organ transplantation is shaped by a utilitarian ethos and a "technocratic approach to healing."[12]

The asymmetry in how the concept of the gift of life plays out for the donor families and for the transplant recipients stems from a denial that donated organs are, at the end of the day, treated as goods or resources that are either good and valuable or bad and worthless. Sharp's ethnographic research found that donor kin "humanize and personify their loved ones through donation" and organ donation is positioned as a way of "making a loved one feel real again," which starkly contrasts with the medical/utilitarian discourse about the organ supply that not only objectifies organs but can sometimes even denigrate them.[13] Sharp writes that over the course of her fieldwork, she sometimes heard surgeons say such things as "I don't want these shitty kidneys."[14] Gift-of-life discourse, on the other hand, is exclusively about saving lives. It can't acknowledge the agony and disappointment when organs have to be discarded because they are essentially objects of no merit and medically unsuitable for transplantation.

In the fantasy version of the transplant story, a donor is someone who was going to "die anyway." Among the faults in this way of thinking is the notion that healthy people "die anyway." I didn't exactly *want* someone to die (it is very difficult, perhaps impossible, to think this), but I didn't take into account that people who "die anyway" are usually not well. Most dying people are not eligible donors for this precise reason. The fact is that most donated livers are not "high quality" and, moreover, the number of transplantable organs is decreasing. One study found that only 29 per cent of donated livers qualified as "high quality."[15]

Death at 6:15

In Shauna's final days, I saw myself as supporting her by refusing to give up or give in, a stance that is echoed throughout the culture of Western biomedicine and seemed to have been adopted by everyone at the hospital.

Fighting death, thwarting death, and keeping death at bay can also be interpreted as forms of denial because of an inability to accept human limitations and mortality. Surgeon Atul Gawande considers medicine's tendency to deny mortality in his insightful book *Being Mortal*. Part of the issue, he argues, is that doctors have difficulty openly acknowledging death with their patients. Instead, they tend to talk about "treatment options" rather than dying, even when death is on the immediate horizon.

Similarly, in her memoir, surgeon Pauline Chen acknowledges that physicians are reluctant to abandon treatment if there is even a "glimmer of hope." She writes that not treating someone or stopping their treatment is seen as "the moral equivalent of giving up," inextricably linked with a sense of failure and defeat. The result is pursuing "hope-driven treatment" at almost any cost.[1] Gawande also acknowledges that treatments are pursued regardless of whether they offer only a "sliver's chance of benefit."[2] While science and medicine are systems of knowledge that privilege rationality, Gawande stresses that hanging on to that sliver's chance stands out as an irrational calculus that, strangely, has become the common thing to do. According to Gawande, doctors have a fear of doing too little, despite evidence that suggests that they routinely do too much. Doing too much has become an accepted part of the medical system.

As Shauna was dying, it wasn't obvious how to contend with the possibility of death when the fantasy of recovery was continually reinforced and played out so dramatically with organ offers. The experience of waiting for a transplant is a particular form of dying that is heavily (very heavily!) steeped in the denial of mortality. Dying was thoroughly off-script; in fact, no one even uttered the word "death." We were anxious about her being "delisted," a technical or bureaucratic term that stood in for dying. We continually described Shauna's situation as a "closing window." We used the word "stable" to describe her ambiguous place on the spectrum between life and death. The moment of death would be a decision to "withdraw support."

Gawande writes, "I knew theoretically that my patients could die, of course, but every instance seemed like a violation, as if the rules we were playing by were broken. I don't know what game I thought this was, but in it we always win."[3] This mentality positions death as a rule infraction. The medical system is built around the possibility of "winning" against the odds, and it fails to prepare patients for outcomes that are "vastly more probable." Gawande writes, "We've created a multitrillion-dollar edifice for dispensing the medical equivalent of lottery tickets – and have only the rudiments of a system to prepare patients for the near-certainty that those tickets will not win."[4]

This orientation towards "winning" means that more and more patients are dying in the ICU following withdrawal of life-sustaining treatments. According to Gawande, "Among patients with chronic diseases who die in the hospital, approximately half are cared for in the ICU in the three days before their death and a third pass at least 10 days in the ICU during the final period of their hospitalisation."[5] In the ICU, patients are in a gray zone between life and death because the distinction between medical care and dying is blurred. When on the "threshold of death," medical technologies can effectively put you "on hold."[6]

Shauna was put on hold. We prolonged Shauna's life and warded off death as much as we possibly could. There was no recognition of the possibility of "excess" treatment, or the limits of acceptability. The trade-off in such cases is that the patient is reduced to a dehumanized state, a "[prisoner] of technical apparatus."[7] Bodily functions and human agency are taken over by machines to which patients are attached by possibly "more than a dozen lines, tubes, or leads."[8] Technology is such an integral part of intensive care; as Lock explains, it is "indispensable not only for supporting the respiration of critically ill patients but also for feeding them, administering medication, and monitoring body functions." Knowledge about the patient's status and condition is also filtered through technology, which, Lock argues, is inherently objectifying. She writes of "the numerous printouts, traces, films, X rays that result from the close monitoring of patients as a kind of 'displacement.' The subjective experience of the patients – their 'personhood' – is unavoidably discounted and replaced by a medical narrative composed of graphs and traces."[9]

Our celebratory attitude about medicine's power to cure disease is apparent in the field of transplantation, but I wasn't fully aware of how the quest to save lives can come with a high cost for patients and families. In Shauna's case, it led to aggressive attempts to repel death even as the prospects of a transplant surgery became riskier and its success more remote and unlikely. As a result, the fantasy of saving her life overrode the reality that she was, in fact, dying. The dismal truth is that her chances were slim, but we refused to see it that way. From the patient's perspective, the stakes of transplantation are high; it is their last and only hope. This is why even if failure is likely, it seems like the superior option to just letting someone die. Any chance was better than no chance at all.

It was this logic that made me never stop to question what was in Shauna's best interest, or my own.

In the early experimental years of transplantation, it was not obvious there was always a balance between providing the best possible care and pursuing treatments that had only a small chance of success. Transplant pioneer Dr Francis Moore asked: "Does the presence of a dying patient justify the doctor taking *any* conceivable step regardless of the degree of hopelessness? ... it gives the impression that physicians and surgeons are adventurers rather than circumspect persons seeking to help the suffering and the dying by the use of hopeful measures. The dying person becomes the object of wildly speculative experiments when he is hopeless and helpless rather than the recipient of discriminating measures carried out on his behalf."[10]

Trailblazing liver transplant surgeon Dr Thomas Starzl thinks, on the other hand, that while such patients may be subjected to aggressive treatments that are unlikely to work, they have at least been given a shot. With reference to pediatric patients, Starzl argues, "Those opposed to trying always claimed that these little creatures [pediatric patients] had been denied the dignity of dying. Their parents believed that they had been given the glory of striving."[11]

When Shauna died, I hardly felt "the glory of striving"; instead, I felt what anthropologist Ruth Behar calls "double sadness." She explains, "Grief stems not simply from the loss of one's beloved but from a consciousness of defeat – the sense that more could have been done, that the struggle ended too soon."[12] Shauna's loss was compounded by grief about the liver transplant itself (that a liver transplant didn't happen felt like a loss in its own right), which stung all the more because, by the standards of being a "good patient," Shauna had tried so hard. We kept up our courage thinking there would be a payoff. We didn't think that she would fight so hard and still lose.

At the time, determination seemed like an integral part of the story. The idea that the volition of the patient can affect prognoses is prevalent in medicine. In the case of cancer, it is frequently framed as a "battle" and "test of moral character," notions Susan Sontag critiques in *Illness as Metaphor*.[13] More recently, Sontag's son David Rieff wrote a memoir about his mother's death from cancer. He explains that despite Sontag's frequently cited critique of illness metaphors, in her own life she herself approached cancer as a "battle."[14] According to Rieff, she viewed her chances of survival as dependent on her willingness to suffer and "her willingness to have the most radical, mutilating treatment." For her, force of will was a weapon. She wanted her entourage, doctors included, to rally around her survival even if it departed from a more "realistic" outlook. Rieff considers that in terminal diagnoses, "There is such thing as too much reality."[15]

Rather than facing the reality of her terminal prognosis, Rieff explains that Sontag looked backward. Her history with cancer was extraordinary. She'd had two previous cancer diagnoses, including metastasized breast cancer in the 1970s that she overcame by seeking out a radical and aggressive therapy. In her experience, pursuing aggressive treatments was the reason why she survived. Thwarting her death on two occasions gave Sontag the sense of "being the author of ... her own disease." Rieff writes, "How, above all, if you struggled to find the right doctors, and braved the most gruesome treatments, can you really say to yourself that none of this really had much to do with why you are still walking on the earth?"[16] In the end, despite her fierce efforts, Sontag died of cancer, leaving Rieff to wonder whether the hubris and the suffering was worth it and whether it would have been better for her to face mortality with more humility and acceptance.

Rieff's memoir resonated with me, particularly his exploration of how focusing exclusively on survival can create ambivalence and regret when death occurs. Part of me feels foolish for not accepting what was obviously coming for my sister.

I once watched a BBC nature documentary with my children that featured a battle between a rattlesnake and a squirrel. The squirrel's strategy was to outsmart and outmanoeuvre the rattlesnake by rubbing some shed snakeskin it found into its fur. It swished its bushy tail from side to side wafting the scent, to make the rattlesnake think, according to the narrator, that a rival was nearby, and creating the illusion of being bigger and more threatening than it really was. The ruse worked. The narrator explained the snake was "confused" by the squirrel's strategy and slithered away. The brave squirrel won.

This astounding glimpse of the natural world impressed my children, but it was easy for me to imagine it ending differently, with the snake striking and devouring the squirrel whole. If the snake had eaten the squirrel, its defences would not have looked so clever and heroic. It may have looked stupid. We imagine that it is valiant to go down with a fight or by taking a wild shot but, depending on the context and the outcome, determined resistance can signify one's failure to accept reality, naïveté, or even lack of wisdom.

I am haunted by what I wrote in the journal post announcing Shauna's pending death because it seems so daft: "We had no idea things were coming to such a bad end." After she died, I posted another message with the help of the hospital chaplain simply noting that her time of death was 6:15 p.m. It also said (in the chaplain's suggested words): "Shauna's suffering is over now and in the loving hands of God."

This was the sudden turnabout in the story, where death is substituted as the salvation that a transplant was supposed to be. The end of "Shauna's suffering" was a dubious way of imposing a semblance of closure.

A seminal study in the mid-1990s found that seeing loved ones connected to tubes and machines and subjecting them to an excess of procedures are reasons why people report a lack of satisfaction with the way their loved ones died. Sharon Kaufman's ethnographic study of ICU death was inspired by this finding.[17] She is intrigued that, despite the general aversion to being "attached to machines," families still accept such strategies when they are offered when faced with the immediate threat of mortality.[18] Kaufman writes, "As long as life-sustaining techniques and pathways exist, they will be wanted and chosen."[19] In her analysis, this is fundamentally because people don't want their loved ones to die.

Ironically, the more "not dying" is pursued, the more the possibility of a "good death" (characterized as being peaceful, easy, comfortable, and without the overuse of technology) fades away. Along with the desire to sustain life, Kaufman argues, "there is simultaneously a loud cry for a kind of dying in which medical intervention is minimized." Kaufman sees this as a paradox of wanting both the best medical treatment and the best death at the same time.[20]

A feature of a "good death" is having the opportunity to face death with courage. A good death involves the "acknowledgement of being on a terminal pathway" with ample time to talk about it and accept it.[21] But modern medicine and healthcare are stacked against the acceptance of death. In a groundbreaking 1965 study, Barney Glaser and Anselm Strauss found that hospital staff will impede awareness of dying at the end of life by "maintaining a fiction" that survival is still possible. Theoretically, "open awareness" of dying is preferred, so that patients and families have the opportunity to be at peace with death before it occurs.[22] But this is not always practised. As Gawande suggests, perhaps no one (physicians, nurses, patients, families) really has the fortitude or the emotional equilibrium to confront death. So its imminence is avoided rather than addressed directly.

There are additional barriers to having open awareness when someone is on life support in the ICU. First of all, they are inaccessible. Many patients are drugged beyond the point of consciousness or coherence. Anthropologist Robert Murphy sees heavy sedation as a form of isolation and a distancing mechanism that makes death a remote experience. He writes, "It is now common in our society for death to come during a drug-induced semi-coma."[23] Dying has become more obscure and inscrutable, and this is alienating for loved ones as well. Lock explains, "New technologies have made death 'invisible' ... an event that the family can neither fully participate in nor verify." Death in the ICU has also been decentralized, in the sense that different body parts can die at different times.[24] In Shauna's case, we were told about multiple organ systems failing, one at a time, though none of this was outwardly obvious.

Moreover, in the ICU, death is not strictly a natural occurrence. It is actively managed and prolonged. According to Kaufman, it's packaged as a "decision." She argues that hospital ICU culture does not treat death like an inevitability or a fact but as a "frame of interpretation," leaving it to the patients and families to "choose" dying. Kaufman's insight is that death in the ICU is a decision about the "switch from life-prolonging moves to making preparations for death moves."[25] With Shauna, this transition was very abrupt. The gap between staving off death and the irrevocable point of death was minuscule.

The night before Shauna died, I didn't stay at the hospital like I usually did. I was exhausted, and the group of Shauna's friends who had become my ad hoc support community determined that I needed a proper night's rest or I was going to lose it completely. My mother decided to stay in my place. My mother had the reputation of being frail both in her physicality and in her demeanour. She is a tiny person. Unlike the rest of the crowd, she wasn't exuberant about the possibility of a victorious ending; she could not sustain that hope. She thought more about defeat than the rest of us, and says now that as a result, she often felt silenced and marginalized.

I think we saw her pessimism as a weakness and so were dismissive of it. I don't think that we could distinguish between accepting that Shauna could die and wanting her to die. They seemed like the same thing. In contrast, my mom believes that she was realistic about the possibility of death the whole time.

That night, she didn't attempt to sleep on the floor of the conference room like I always did but instead settled into a recliner in the ICU waiting room. There were two recliners in the waiting room. They were fiercely coveted because all the other chairs were lined up around the perimeter of the room and bolted to the ground, with thin padding, straight backs, and armrests that prevented stretching out or any other attempts at getting comfortable. A recliner needed to be staked out by vigilantly watching for the rare occasion one was vacated, at which point someone would have to spring upon it as quickly as possible to make sure it was occupied by one of our group for the rest of the day.

The ICU nurse was usually available first thing in the morning to let us know how Shauna's night had been and give updates on her "stability." So I got up early and headed to the hospital. I was allowed into the ward right away. This is what I remember: I was in the hallway outside Shauna's room putting on a gown and gloves when the nurse, a new one I had never met before, came up to me and said, "Oh, you don't need to gown and glove. Shauna's been delisted for transplant."

The scene that followed could have been directed by John Cassavetes. As a filmmaker, Cassavetes is known for directing emotionally wrought performances, perhaps most notably that of Gena Rowlands in *A Woman Under the Influence* (1974), which has been described as an intense, vivid, and chaotic portrayal of a character whose world is crumbling.[26] I don't remember exactly what happened next. I know that there was shouting. I know I accused the nurse of not having a fucking clue what she was talking about. The commotion was quickly quelled by the head nurse, who immediately saw that the hostility between me and that "Shauna is delisted" nurse was irreparable. She switched her to the far end of the ward where we wouldn't cross paths again (I wanted her to go to hell, or worse) and assigned another nurse to care for Shauna for the day.

I called the transplant coordinator nurse. She assured me that she had heard nothing about Shauna being delisted, but later in the day there was going to be a family meeting. I requested the presence of the hepatologist Dr P., who was tied up in his clinic that day with appointments but available later in the afternoon. I needed him there because I trusted him the most. His opinion was the only one that mattered to me. The family meeting was with Dr P., the transplant coordinator nurse and the rest of the transplant team, the ICU docs, and Shauna's ICU nurse for the day. There were boxes of Kleenex on the table. I guess we knew what they were going to say.

It was unanimous that life support should be withdrawn. Transplant was no longer possible.

We had been warned about the possibility of other organ systems failing, and neither Shauna's heart (low blood pressure and erratic rhythms) nor her lungs were in good shape anymore. In combination with her failed liver and kidneys, this meant she had "multi-system organ failure" (the cause of death written on her death certificate). We had known about the possibility of infection, given her fragility, and we were told she had an infection too.

We gathered around her bed with the ICU nurse who was going to turn the ventilator off and remove the ventilator tube. There was no process of dying to witness. There truly was no life left in her. It was instantaneous. Without the ventilator, Shauna didn't take a single breath.

There was, however, a shocking sense of rupture and ugliness and brutality to the suddenness of the break. Maybe I was expecting more of a soothing letting go, or a drifting away, but it was like she had just been sucked out of an airplane at lightning speed, snapped into oblivion. Her fast disappearance felt empty to me. I wish death felt more lush or dense. I yearned for something consoling like peace or transcendence, which I found a bit in the bone structure of her face that was so delicate, and in her clear smooth skin.

Foundationally, I collapsed (a friend noted that part of me had died too). I felt hollow, like my most inner part was suspended and had no essence, sensation, or physicality. I went blank. Feelings seared straight through me without landing in my body.

My mother wanted Shauna spared the indignity of being sent to the hospital morgue, so we waited with her in her room for the funeral home staff to arrive with their black suits, formal demeanour, and synthetic sympathy. In the meantime, another *persona non grata*, the attending ICU doctor, came in to "pronounce death" (a redundancy) and sign the death certificate, a bureaucratic intrusion and gesture of ordinariness that clashed with our monumental loss.

Everything about it felt wrong. Shauna's death was essentially a message received in a boardroom, a setting that is far too staid for the intensity of life-and-death matters. It's appropriate, though, for the delivery of grave news and making a logical case. Shauna's condition had been "managed" and "controlled," but now it had become "unmanageable" and "out of control." The doctors were clear they had no more tools, tricks, or magic. Everyone at the table said so, and everything collapsed in that boardroom meeting into a meaningless gnarl of futility.

Bob Dylan recorded a song in the late 1970s called "Señor (Tales of Yankee Power)." Dylan experts have grouped it with his "south-of-the-border adventure songs," replete with moral lessons, religious symbolism, political critique, and tearing down illusions. I think about that boardroom only at the very end, when Dylan sings about overturning tables because, ultimately, there are no answers. We aren't waiting for anything.

The idea of overturning tables is my fantasy version of what happened. In that boardroom I sat still and wept, but it would have been preferable to stand up and flip the tables over. Willie Nelson's cover of the song is even better because his voice is a mournful and gentle counterpoint to my vision of trashing the boardroom.

The Story of MELD

Every year thousands of patients are listed for a liver transplant. Approximately 10 to 25 per cent of those people become "delisted." Some succumb to "waitlist mortality"; others are removed for being too sick to survive the procedure.[1] In the US, eight people waiting for a liver transplant die every day. This translates into one in six dying on liver transplant waitlists every year.[2] In 2004, the year Shauna died, in the US region where Shauna resided there were 448 liver transplants and 168 deaths on the waitlist. Eleven of those deaths were patients between the ages of eighteen and thirty-four. Shauna was one of these eleven people.[3]

I look at these numbers and think: Why wasn't my sister among the much larger pool of 448 transplanted patients? Is this an unanswerable question about why bad things happen by chance? I would never argue against luck and misfortune having a hand in all aspects of life. But honestly, what were the odds? Now, when I hear that some kind of unlikely awful thing has happened, it rings familiar. That figures. Fists clenched. That's how the world works.

Waiting for a transplant is inherently a passive experience. This clashes with a general sense that you shouldn't just passively wait for anything in life. Losers do that.

Successful people are proactive. But there was nothing we could have done to expedite or guarantee the transplant. We sometimes heard the advice to "pressure the docs" or "lean on the docs," as though a more aggressive attitude was required – that the doctors could do more to procure a liver donor, and we could forcefully insist upon it. But it didn't work like that. You had to wait your turn.

Our family, as a general rule, didn't lean on people, pressure them, or game systems; even being assertive didn't sit right with our family principles and moral system. Shauna and I were reared as do-gooders. When we were girls, our mother brought us along with her to volunteer at the Ronald McDonald House, a large home near the university hospital that had been converted to a boarding house for out-of-town and financially-in-need families of critically ill children. Our mother did housework there and Shauna and I helped with chores, like we did at home. The chores we did there were not that significant – tidying, sweeping, dusting – but this ethos of doing things for the benefit of others extended to the way we saw organ donation. We embraced the idea that it was a selfless act of generosity. We would wait our turn, and it would happen the way we thought it was supposed to – receiving a generous gift from a benevolent stranger.

In our society, we're accustomed to the idea of using privilege and power to get what we want. Organ transplantation is hardly exempt from this. The black-market organ trade is a stark example of the way that racial and economic inequalities are exploitable, and have been exploited, by transplantation. But there are other less egregious ways of gaming the system. In the US, patients can be listed at more than one transplant centre at a time to increase their chances. This is an advantage that only wealthier people have, because it involves travel costs, additional living expenses, and paying out of pocket for services at multiple transplant centres (such as doctor's visits, tests, and evaluations), because any insurance provider would most likely only cover their cost at a single centre, not two or more. Deceased liver transplant recipient and Apple CEO Steve Jobs was listed at multiple centres. He was a California resident but he was transplanted in Tennessee, leading to questions about whether or not he really got his transplant fair and square.[4]

There is more context, however, for understanding who gets transplants and who does not, namely how the waiting list works and the specifics of liver allocation policy. Doctors determine medically (and psychologically) suitable candidates: those who will likely benefit from transplantation without having other medical issues and complications that would cancel out those benefits. In other words, there is a utility benchmark for being vetted into candidacy. Once in that lucky pool, candidates are then prioritized according to who is most likely to die.

It wasn't always like this. In the 1960s and 1970s, transplant programs in the US made allocation decisions with no formal guidelines. One surgeon states that "procedures and policies were largely left to the conscience and common sense of transplant physicians and surgeons involved."[5] This approach came to an end in 1984, when the US Congress passed the National Organ Transplantation Act (NOTA), which established the Organ Procurement and Transplantation Network (OPTN). The OPTN banned discrimination based on race, sex, and class, and discouraged giving weight to social criteria like age and lifestyle.[6] Their goal was to centralize the administration of a single national procurement and allocation system. In 1986, the United Network of Organ Sharing (UNOS), a non-profit private organization, was given a contract to establish a national organ distribution network and oversee allocation. Since then, in the US, allocation is determined by UNOS policies.

For the first ten years (1986–96), UNOS decided that liver allocation should be based on the level and location of care. Hospitalized patients in the intensive care unit had the highest priority, followed by hospitalized patients on the regular floor, and further down the list were those receiving outpatient care. The liver transplant community questioned the fairness of this system. There was concern about the potentially arbitrary nature of ranking patients by the location of care. Specifically, physicians could manipulate it to give some patients more priority over others by hospitalizing patients or placing them in ICU just because they could.[7] It was not a rigorous way of determining the actual medical status of waitlisted patients.

In 1996, a consensus conference mandated that the Child–Pugh–Turcotte (CPT) score be used along with location of care for liver allocation. The CPT score is based on objective markers of liver health, serum albumin and serum bilirubin, and prothrombin time, which is how long it takes your blood to clot, also a sign of liver health because clotting proteins are made in the liver. The CPT score also included two so-called subjective criteria: the severity of ascites and encephalopathy.[8] Wait time was used as an ordering tool for candidates with similar medical status. However, questions about fairness persisted. One critique was that the subjective criteria (ascites and encephalopathy) of the CPT score were open to interpretation by individual physicians and too difficult to standardize. Another critique concerned wait time as an ordering tool and the "first come, first served logic," because the point at which a patient is first listed for transplant does not necessarily correspond to the severity of their liver disease. The patients added early to the waitlist are those who have higher access to medical care (often from a higher socioeconomic demographic), so those who entered the list later because of lack of access to medical care were at a disadvantage, exacerbating health disparities.[9]

The desired solution was a more objective and systematic definition of disease severity that could be used as countrywide criteria to rank liver transplants candidates.[10] In 1999, the OPTN formed the Liver Disease Severity Score Committee, tasked with developing a model to assess disease severity using only "biochemical derangements from liver failure."[11] Rather than reinvent the wheel, they looked to the Model for End-Stage Liver Disease (MELD) that had already been developed at the Mayo Clinic. MELD is an algorithm that calculates a patient's INR (international normalization ratio for prothrombin time, a standardized way to measure how long it takes your blood to clot), serum creatinine (a measurement of kidney function), and serum bilirubin (a measurement of liver function), and results in a score between zero and forty. Researchers tested whether MELD could be used for predicting waitlist mortality for transplant candidates with chronic liver disease. Using five different data sets, MELD was validated as effective at predicting three-month waiting list mortality and was found to be generalizable to a heterogeneous group of patients, including those who were hospitalized or ambulatory and had cholestatic or non-cholestatic liver disease (the former is caused by bile flow blockage while the latter is not).[12] The MELD score was adopted in the US on 28 February 2002 as the liver allocation tool for chronic liver disease candidates. MELD was adopted in Canada in 2004.

MELD is an important milestone. It was perceived as a data-driven policy change that ensured livers were distributed to the "sickest first" according to "readily available, reproducible and objective data."[13] Shauna's MELD score was an intense preoccupation for us throughout her period of waiting for a transplant. MELD is seared into my brain so deeply that, to this day, it randomly appears in my dreams. We were acutely aware that the MELD score largely determines who does or doesn't get transplanted. It also changes what it means to wait. In general, time can be a significant factor when it comes to waiting. Spending more time waiting can make you feel closer to whatever it is you are waiting for. But liver transplantation doesn't work this way. You move up the list as your MELD score worsens. Candidates' lab results are reported on a set schedule and the list is configured accordingly; candidates move up or down not only based on their own scores but also according to the scores of other candidates, and in relation to how many candidates have been transplanted, have been delisted, or have died. The top of the list is no longer fixed, and no one is simply waiting to get there. The only way to the top is according to "disease severity."

After Shauna died, I saw that in pages of her journal from early 2004 she was transcribing the weekly lists that ranked waitlisted patients at the two regional liver transplant centres: Duke and the University of North Carolina (UNC). Shauna was listed at Duke, but as livers become available in the region, candidates at both Duke and UNC were given equal consideration. The transcribed lists show the number of patients per her blood type (type A) and MELD ranges. She herself is somewhere in those anonymous lists among the dozens of patients in the eleven to eighteen range, too low for transplant to be a realistic possibility. Effectively, at this point she wasn't waiting for a transplant but waiting to get sicker. For this reason, her low MELD score wasn't reassuring. It just created anxiety

Tracking statistics while waiting, using MELD data.

about her getting sicker, knowing that simply time on the list would have no bearing on her chances.

Shauna's transposition of publicly available data into her private journal was a form of sense-making. The lists are a genre of narrativity where meaning is derived from what they are not explicitly saying, only hinting. It's like telling her story through found footage. I note that on 23 January, she drew a flower in the margin. On the following page she jotted down a reference to a journal article, "Distributing Scarce Livers: The Moral Reasoning of the General Public," published in *Social Science and Medicine*. She summarizes transplant data for patients

> Questions
> ① Post TX exacerbation of IBD?
> ② Cholecystectomy (gallbladder removal) at TX?
>   - roux-en-y procedure?
> ③ Statistical significance of the difference between MELD scores -- is the supposed "continuity" of the model an illusion?
>
> Duke Transplants (Cadaveric) - Type A
> Jan-Nov '03   2002   2001   2000
>   10   14   18   13
>   average = 15/year
> 365/15 = 24.3 days between transplants
>   (type A) on average.
> ⇒ (24.3) × (spot on list) = average waiting time
>   if 9th → 219 days (≈ 7 months)
>
> UNC Transplants (Cadaveric) - Type A
> Jan-Nov '03   2002   2001   2000
>   17   20   16   26
>   average = 20.6/year
> 365/20.6 = 17.7 days between transplants
>
> Combined Duke/UNC Type A transplants
> 15 + 20.6 = 35.6 transplants (A)/year
> 365/35.6 = 10.25 days between transplants on average.
>
> ⇒ if 20th on combined list
>   (10.25) × 20 = 205 days average waiting time.

Shauna's questions for her healthcare team, followed by her arithmetic forecast of her wait for a liver transplant based on average number of days between liver transplants (type A) at Duke and UNC. Her projected wait is 205 days. Though undated, this entry is likely from February 2004. The 205-day projection roughly aligns with when the chapter "Die Waiting" begins.

with PSC, like her, does a rough but clearly presented calculation of average wait times based on blood type and the number of days between transplants, and writes a list of three questions, including "Statistical significance of the difference between MELD scores – is the supposed 'continuity' of the model an illusion?"

In a way, these lists convey so little information that they are almost vacuous, unrevealing like the MELD score itself. MELD doesn't predict when you will get a transplant. Neither does it say very much about your "disease severity" because it has nothing to do with your functional status, symptom burden, or the pain and distress you are feeling. Even though it is presented as a "prognostic score," it hardly provides a meaningful prognosis.

Each number (zero to forty) corresponds to a statistic of ninety-day mortality risk: that is, the likelihood that you will die in the next three months. For example, a MELD of thirty means a ninety-day mortality rate of 65 per cent. While statistically reliable, it doesn't translate into knowing exactly what to expect. It just describes, as all statistics do, the chances in general.[14]

Statistics leave patients with very little to go on. A measure of probability based on aggregated data is, as Ann Jurecic argues, "not a representation of one's future." She writes, "While general populations can be described with probabilities, the life of an individual cannot."[15] MELD has nothing to do with the real lives of actual patients; it is a tool for measuring and quantifying mortality as a basis for objective decision-making. Current health policy prefers this kind of quantification and the application of rational technical rules. This orientation is consistent with the idea of evidence-based medicine (EBM), namely that healthcare standards should be based on generalizable and universal research evidence.[16]

Shauna, given her training in economics, was partial to objective measures and believed that the MELD policy was a good thing. We had superficial conversations about it back when she was first listed for a transplant. She saw it as an improvement over the previous system because it eliminated the subjective judgment of physicians in the prioritization of liver transplant candidates. I remember her explaining to me that the MELD system was designed to create equality for all candidates precisely because it only compares lab scores.

The perception that MELD promotes fairness and equality demonstrates the influence of liberalism in public institutions like health care. Political theorist Iris Marion Young describes this as "equality conceived as sameness," reflecting the liberal idea that commonalities can transcend particularities and differences and give rise to universal standards – like basic human rights, or simply the idea that everybody should be treated the same way.[17] Treating all patients the same way is a pillar of EBM. It assumes that evidence that applies to a large sample can also be applied in each individual case. Critics of EBM, however, argue that more complex health experiences are being reduced to simple numerical indicators that are easier for management to administer and compatible with "audit culture," but are highly decontextualized.[18] Greenhalgh and her fellow investigators go on to note that patients are not "fixed entities" and suggest that in a more patient-centred approach to medicine, the focus would not be just on mean values but also on the way that "illness as lived" can differ from "the disease or risk state in the evidence-based guideline."[19] Surgeon Pauline Chen notes that as a "professional method of coping," physicians can even turn away from interactions with patients, "concentrating instead on 'treatment algorithms' for their 'disease progression'" and treating them as "cases in the context of objective data" rather than as patients in the here and now.[20]

In the MELD system, all patients are ranked according to the same measures, premised on the idea that there is a standardized experience of end-stage liver disease that renders all patients comparable. MELD played a role in shaping Shauna's trajectory because it is narrowly focused on only three clinical markers and does not take into consideration others that may also be poor prognostic indicators. Studies have suggested that portal hypertension, refractory ascites, and hepatorenal syndrome are underweighted by MELD for determining mortality risk.[21] These are all complications Shauna had.

MELD policy as it was initially conceived was flawed. Some of the flaws in the MELD system have resulted in policy changes since it was first implemented. The MELD system today is different than it was at the time that Shauna died. Notably, in 2016 the MELD score was officially changed to include serum sodium in the calculation for all transplant patients. MELD is now MELD-Na. This change resulted from studies that showed that low serum sodium, or hyponatremia, was an independent predictor of mortality in liver transplant patients, and that including sodium scores improved MELD's accuracy in predicting mortality.[22] In 2004, Shauna fell through the cracks of an untested system of allocation that didn't take into consideration hyponatremia's strong link to pretransplant mortality.

There's no way to know if MELD-Na would have really made a difference in Shauna's case because there were also other features of MELD that were stacked against her. One aspect of the MELD stem that reduced her chances *by design* was the designation of status 1A to a specific cohort of patients. As the name connotes, these are the highest-priority patients. They don't even calculate a MELD score for these patients, who default to the top of the list. To qualify as status 1A you must meet the criteria of "fulminant liver failure," defined as "the onset of hepatic encephalopathy [when toxins build up in the blood and affect brain function] within 56 days of the first signs or symptoms of liver disease." Status 1A patients cannot have a pre-existing diagnosis of liver disease unless they are a recent recipient of a (failed) transplant experiencing "primary non-function of a transplanted whole liver within 7 days of transplant." They also must be in the ICU, either on a ventilator or on continuous hemodialysis.[23] Shauna, in the rapidly terminal phase of her chronic illness, did not qualify as a status 1A patient. Though death was imminent for her as much as it was for any status 1A patient on a ventilator and dialysis, she was ranked lower on the list because of the history of her disease.

Shauna always referred to status 1A patients somewhat wryly as "people who take too much Tylenol," whether this happened intentionally or accidentally, as a result of not reading the label correctly or at all, or misinterpreting the dosage. Almost a quarter of status 1A patients have acetaminophen toxicity; it is the most common cause of fulminant liver failure (most other status 1A patients are in the category of non-acetaminophen toxicity or have immediate post-graft failure).[24] Status 1A patients are rare (fewer than 1 per cent). Shockingly, the day before Shauna died the transplant coordinator nurse very gently told us that there were not one but two status 1A patients in the region. Effectively, it made Shauna third on the list, which might as well have been the very bottom.

When Shauna died, her MELD had reached forty. Patients with MELDs between thirty-six and forty and status 1A patients have no difference in waitlist mortality despite status 1A patients having automatic higher priority.[25] Another study found that 11 per cent of status 1A patients "are not as critically ill as imagined" and recommended that status 1A patients be stratified into high-risk and low-risk classes.[26] Of course I don't know whether these status 1A patients lived, or died like Shauna, but the nurse was letting us know that an organ offer wouldn't be likely. The thought of those status 1A patients is still a weird fixation that fills me with despair.

As I was reading more about MELD, I learned there was another group of patients who were significantly advantaged in the early MELD era: those with liver cancer known as hepatocellular carcinoma (HCC). From the start, one of the challenges for implementing MELD was how to include HCC patients. MELD measures risk of mortality from liver disease, whereas HCC patients are at risk of dying from the "progression of their malignancy."[27] For this reason, the liver transplant community agreed that a MELD score would not accurately predict mortality risk for HCC patients. So HCC patients have *allocated* (not calculated) MELD scores and a policy was adopted to allow standardized exception points for those candidates. These exception points were initially far too high, and HCC patients were overprioritized for transplantation. The number of exception points was reduced in 2003 and even further reduced in 2005. Ten years later, in 2015, the exception points were reduced even more, because HCC patients were still overprioritized.[28]

The excessive priority for HCC liver transplant candidates was a huge disadvantage for ESLD patients waiting for a transplant, especially in the early years of MELD (2002–05) when Shauna was waitlisted. When MELD was first introduced, nearly three-quarters of HCC patients received transplants within the first three months of being listed (!!!). They had a significantly decreased risk of waitlist mortality and increased odds of transplantation compared to patients with end-stage liver disease (ranked with "native MELD scores").[29] Some have argued this is "not surprising" given that the policies surrounding exception points were not evidence based and "no clinical data from actual transplant candidates were used to make these decisions" at the time.[30]

Even more significantly, I learned that recent research indicates there is systemic sex/gender bias in the MELD system. MELD has increased this disparity amongst liver transplant recipients – more men are getting liver transplants than women. In fact, MELD has produced an increase in waitlist mortality for female liver transplant candidates. The issues that contribute to this disparity are not well understood but possibly include body size and MELD's incorrect assessment of disease severity, especially related to the use of creatinine as a measure of kidney function.[31] Creatinine is a waste product made by muscles, filtered through the kidneys. Women typically have lower creatinine levels than men because they have less muscle mass. Other researchers have pointed to gender bias in the selection process of transplant candidates.[32]

It is true that more men suffer from end-stage liver disease than women and therefore that the prevalence of diseases for which transplantation may be indicated is not equally distributed between women and men. For example, cirrhosis is more common in men than in women.[33] Overall, fewer women are listed for transplant – they represent about 36.1 per cent of patients waiting.[34] However, the concerning issue is that the introduction of MELD has reduced waitlist mortality for men and increased it for women.[35] The first study that looked at the impact of race and gender on waitlist mortality in the MELD era, using data from 2002–07, found that women had a higher waitlist mortality: 23.7 per cent of women die on waitlist vs 21.9 per cent of men.[36] More recent studies have found this gap has widened since then. A study in 2018 found the difference to be 22 per cent waitlist mortality for women and 18 per cent for men.[37] A 2020 study using data from 2013–18 found that 41 per cent of patients who die on waitlist are women and 59 per cent are men; when these percentages are adjusted to reflect the distribution of men and women on the waitlist, this represents an 8.6 per cent greater risk of waitlist mortality for women. The same study found that women are 14.4 per cent less likely to receive a deceased donation.[38] Studies have also found that women have a higher mortality compared to men with the same MELD scores, specifically a 19 per cent higher risk of waitlist mortality.[39]

Despite the fact that MELD was intended to be unbiased, twenty years of data shows that there *is* a consistent bias against women. In 2023, a new version of MELD was adopted to reduce sex disparities. MELD 3.0, as it is called, now includes sex and albumin as variables in addition to giving less weight to creatinine and more weight to bilirubin.[40] The researchers who developed the new algorithm estimated "that the new score would reclassify approximately 9% of the people who died while waiting and reduce at least 20 waitlist deaths per year."[41] While I don't have her lab values to prove it, I can't help but situate Shauna as one of the individuals who would have benefited from MELD 3.0 (one whose score would have been higher in this new algorithm, increasing her opportunity for transplant) and think that she is a textbook example of why MELD 3.0 is an improvement, especially for women.

The original MELD did not represent disease severity accurately across different diagnoses. The initial study that validated MELD as a predictor of mortality overrepresented men, particularly white men with hepatitis C,[42] which is more likely to lead to renal impairment than cholestatic and autoimmune liver diseases, which more women have,[43] including Shauna whose renal function was good up until her rapid decline. Her serum creatinine was the main reason why her MELD score had never previously been high enough to reach the top of the list.

Looking at Shauna's experiences through the history of MELD shows that her chances of an optimistic outcome were hindered. It makes it *not* surprising that Shauna died. This almost feels like a betrayal, like the system wasn't on her side.

A couple weeks after Shauna died, our friend Katy and I took a short trip to New York City. We stayed with friends in Brooklyn but spent our days wandering Manhattan briskly and aimlessly, wrapped up in scarves and wearing gloves. (I also stayed in bed quite a bit – smoked marijuana in bed, drank beer in bed, and looked at a pile of *Life* magazines from the 1930s and 1940s in bed.) As I remember it, the sky was fiercely blue and the air was crisp, cold, and refreshing, and hit the right notes in me. I was temporarily buoyed by the flow and fullness of New York, a contrast to the idleness of the previous months spent waiting in the hospital in Durham. It was a fortifying trip.

To get to New York, Katy and I drove from Durham to Richmond, Virginia, and took the Amtrak. We were running late and nearly missed the train. As we barrelled through Richmond to get to the station, I saw a large, single-storey building with a sign on the lawn: UNOS, the national headquarters of the United Network of Organ Sharing, the organization that manages the US organ transplant system and determines donation and transplantation policies. There it was.

In retrospect, I was probably mistaken. The UNOS headquarters is indeed in Richmond, Virginia. However, a Google search shows that it looks nothing like the building I saw from the car window. From the images on the internet, the real UNOS is a four-storey building with extensive landscaping, surrounded by a memorial garden. But the steely cynicism triggered by "seeing" UNOS still feels so real to me. In fact, that four-storey UNOS building was only constructed in 2003, and the memorial garden wasn't completed in 2004. It's possible that day in December 2004, I saw the *old* UNOS headquarters, an abandoned building, an empty piece of real estate. A deserted UNOS fits with how I thought of UNOS at the time: a sham and a scam, *caveat emptor*. If there had been more time, I would have wanted to stop and throw a brick at the old UNOS in fury.

Failure

After Shauna died, I remember a brief exchange with her hepatologist, Dr P., in the hospital hallway. I knew he was devastated because Shauna had been a dear patient of his for several years. He acknowledged it was a shame that a transplant had never happened, then added something vague and disparaging about liver transplantation as a "rough and ready" solution as he scanned his hospital ID card on the wall next to where we were standing and disappeared behind a locked door. It was a jarring thought to part on. Why would he describe a liver transplant as "rough and ready"? The dictionary defines "rough and ready" as "simple but good enough to use"; also as "not having polite or fancy skills but ready and able to do what needs to be done." This was so confusing.

After losing Shauna, I don't think Dr P. thought there was anything he could say that would have really been consoling.[1] I don't suspect he thought that describing liver transplantation as "rough and ready" could cut through the awkwardness and difficulty of knowing that it seemed to us that he, and all the other doctors, had let us down; indeed, I don't doubt that my sister's medical team harboured their own sense of failure. But reframing a black and white solution (the way I saw a transplant) as a flawed or limited option was something I was much too vulnerable to consider.

My perception of transplant had always been very naïve, almost childish. Shauna was diagnosed with autoimmune hepatitis in 1986 when she was eleven and I was ten. Over the course of the next few years, she developed inflammatory bowel diseases (Crohn's and ulcerative colitis) and then primary sclerosing cholangitis (PSC), an autoimmune disease that hardens the bile ducts. One autoimmune disease creates a predisposition for others, and this cluster of diagnoses was not outside the norm in gastroenterology. When Shauna's PSC was diagnosed in 1994, she was a nineteen-year-old university student. Her prognosis was uncertain, but it was agreed that eventually she would need a liver transplant. Maybe in ten years.

In the mid-1990s, I hardly knew anything about liver transplantation. I assumed that it was a well-established procedure that saved lives. I believed that a liver transplant would be successful and Shauna's health problems would become less severe and debilitating, if not instantly disappear. I had unquestioned faith that life-saving biomedical technologies relieved suffering – it seemed obvious in the case of organ transplantation. It would mean "liberation from disease."[2]

Years after Shauna died, I cracked open *Transplant: From Myth to Reality* by Dr Nicholas Tilney, one of the many books of hers that I kept after she died. Published by Yale University Press in 2002 and written by "an international authority on organ transplantation," the book presents an account of "the development of this exciting field." I learned that the first experimental liver transplants (on dogs) in the mid-1950s went very badly. Early experiments with humans were rife with post-operative complications like uncontrollable bleeding, infection, bile leaks, and obstructions, if the patients didn't die from shock during surgery. These challenges stemmed from the liver's functional complexity, so there was a need for innovations and refinements in surgical techniques to avoid losing patients to operative complications.[3]

In terms of success rate, liver transplantation had a terrible start. By the mid-1970s there had been a total of 130 liver transplants, but only 12 recipients survived. Given these "marginal results," Tilney admits that there was "little enthusiasm" for liver transplantation.[4] According to him, the field was driven by "a handful of single-minded surgical-scientists" who "labored to wrest the technically demanding transplantation of these complex organs from the realm of total failure."[5] Chief among them was Thomas Starzl, considered to be the father of liver transplantation, the first to execute a successful human liver transplant in 1967.

In Starzl's memoir *The Puzzle People*, he emphasizes that his work in liver transplantation was not initially regarded with much esteem. Nor was it lucrative. Early in his career, working at the University of Miami, Starzl set up a lab in a garage across from the hospital, content with its basic amenities – running water and a central drain. Research funds were so limited he was required to maintain this laboratory out of his own pocket. He experimented using dogs from the city pound that were cared for by his wife, and cast-off or "borrowed" equipment from the hospital. Starzl moved on to Northwestern University, where in 1959, he was awarded a prestigious scholarship to do research, with a stipend of $6,000 per year. This allowed him to work in the lab "all day everyday." Still, he recalls that money was so tight that when the head of the medical school of the University of Western Virginia visited him in Chicago, his wife cooked them a rabbit Starzl had stolen from a laboratory.

In the 1960s and 1970s, survival for all patients given organ transplants was minimal. Kidney transplantation had shown the biggest strides and the most promise, but even Tilney summarizes those early decades as "isolated, usually hopeless ... attempts of a few innovative surgeons to preserve by any means available an occasional patient dying from nonfunctioning kidneys."[6] He describes a global convention in 1963 that analyzed all available clinical information on kidney transplantation and found dismal results: 52 per cent of grafts from related living donors had resulted in death and 81 per cent of those who had received kidneys from cadaveric donors had died. Of those who received kidneys from cadavers, only 4 per cent had lived for more than a year, while two-thirds of kidney graft recipients died within months.[7] Due to this high mortality, there was doubt that kidney transplantation could be widely implemented. Similarly, in the late 1960s, Starzl deemed liver transplantation "feasible but impractical" and questioned whether it was "worth this much trouble to save so few people."[8]

One of the factors that changed transplantation's trajectory was a bill passed by the US Congress in 1972 that allowed patients with kidney disease to be funded under Medicare and receive a kidney transplant as a therapeutic option. This support resulted from extensive lobbying by patients, physicians, and industry.[9] Transplant surgeon Barry Kahan describes the government decision to fund kidney transplantation as "amazing ... not only because the results were not worthy of it, nor was transplantation in 1972 prepared for this imprimatur. Not only were organ recovery systems primitive, but one-year success rates of transplantation were 60 per cent at best."[10]

With the backing of the government, kidney transplantation was fast-tracked to becoming a standard treatment.

While on the one hand this makes progress in transplantation seem smooth and linear, it also underscores that it was contingent on circumstances that, in retrospect, seem irregular. It wasn't driven by science but rather by consensus about the *desirability* of transplants: a consensus that wasn't entirely rooted in reality. Tilney notes that therapeutic limitations of kidney transplantation had been downplayed by the lobbying effort. Starzl thinks this occurred to the point that "the integrity of the field" was nearly compromised. Overly optimistic claims about kidney transplantation floated around, which, according to Starzl, "were deceptive at best and potentially fraudulent at worst."[11] The overstatement of success and the lack of transparency about mortality meant that the public (via the media) received a more optimistic perspective about transplantation than was warranted. Tilney believes that the general public embraced the promise of transplantation because it was thirsty for optimism. He writes, "In contrast to the continuing national crises, disruptions, and self-doubts of that period, apparently positive medical 'miracles' caught the public interest and improved its mood."[12]

Public optimism about organ transplantation was particularly fuelled by the media spotlight on heart transplantation in the late 1960s. The first doctor to perform a human-to-human heart transplant was the South African cardiologist Dr Christiaan Barnard. This feat was celebrated by a *Time* magazine cover story (15 December 1967) and kicked off a spate of sensationalistic media coverage.[13] Anthropologist Margaret Lock argues that the publicity around heart transplantation fostered a distorted, overly optimistic perception of its potential. For her this is exemplified by a published photograph of Philip Blaiberg, the South African third recipient of a heart transplant, swimming in the ocean as a testament to his recovery and good health. The truth was that Blaiberg never walked again after his surgery. Lock reveals that "for the photograph he had to be taken down to the water's edge in a wheelchair, carried into the ocean, photographed, and then hauled out again." Blaiberg only lived for nineteen months and fifteen days with his new heart before he died. The photograph, therefore, was a contrived representation of medical triumph that masked the limited benefits of heart transplantation at that time.[14]

In reading about the history of transplantation, I wasn't anticipating that I would find that my own overly optimistic, fantasy-tinged view had so much concordance with the historical context of transplantation, and with the way such a skewed perception is almost baked into the field. A tendency to confuse the success of the procedure with its potential gives it a distinct ontological status as both real and illusory at the same time. My own understanding of transplantation as the be all and end all had been a blurring of fact and fantasy, a fixation on its unrealized capacity. This theme seems to run through this medical domain. For example, "Together we will turn transplantation into a cure" is the mission of the Canadian Donation and Transplantation Research Program.[15] On the surface, it's a nice optimistic message. But now I am attuned to its oblique admission that transplantation is *not*, in fact, a cure.

The major impediment to realizing transplantation's potential as a cure is graft intolerance (the host body's rejection of foreign tissue). Without inducing tolerance, transplantation has no chance of being viable. Tilney describes early methods used on kidney transplant recipients to overcome the immune barrier that were ghastly and extreme, such as total-body irradiation. Patients received a massive dose of radiation "as they lay curled on the floor on a mattress within the circumference of the beam."[16] Although the intent was to increase recipients' tolerance of grafts, everyone died from the total suppression of their immune defences. Thereafter radiation treatment was reduced to intermittent small doses, and cortisone was administered to reverse episodes of rejection.

The evolution of organ transplantation depended on gaining more understanding of the complexity of the immune system. Nobel Prize–winning microbiologist Peter Medawar undertook pioneer work in immunology in the 1960s and 1970s, which greatly influenced the development of organ transplantation. Medawar, who happened to be "too tall to serve in the army" during World War II, began experimenting on the treatment of burns. He studied the way "the body discriminated between its own and foreign tissue" and the rejection of skin grafts.[17] Medawar eventually identified the cellular components of the immune system (lymphocytes) and focused his attention on the role of antibodies.[18] He clearly articulated rejection as an immune-system response and defined "tolerance" as "a state in which an animal or even a patient can be made selectively unresponsive to the antigens of a given graft, while the remainder of immunological defense mechanisms remain intact."[19] Tilney argues that it was Medawar's precise definitions of tolerance and rejection that guided the development of organ transplantation.[20]

One of the first immunosuppression drugs was azathioprine, which was effective at delaying and reducing rejection. However, there were also numerous negative side effects of immunosuppressants, such that Tilney notes the "treatment sometimes appeared worse than the original disease" and led to poor outcomes in terms of long-term survival.[21] The most significant clinical advancement was the discovery of a new drug – cyclosporine A – in the late 1970s. It was derived from fungi that field botanists with the Swiss pharmaceutical company Sandoz had collected from "a bleak highland plateau in Norway ... and a valley in Wisconsin." Cyclosporine had impressive immunosuppressive abilities as well as a lack of toxicity and rapidly boosted post-transplant survival.[22] It was a "game changer," becoming the standard treatment for transplant patients and significantly expanding the horizons of transplantation.

Cyclosporine was a major milestone for liver transplantation. As it increased post-transplant survival, Starzl saw an opportunity to bolster liver transplantation by converting its status from "experimental" to "therapeutic." Meeting with the US surgeon general in 1982, Starzl initiated plans for a congressional hearing in 1983 to determine whether liver transplantation was an acceptable medical service now that cyclosporine could treat rejection. Starzl had transplanted 120 livers between 1963 and 1979, but only thirty-three patients (27.5 per cent) had survived for twelve months. Comparatively, he transplanted forty livers in 1980 and 1981 using cyclosporine, and twenty-eight patients (70 per cent) were alive twelve months later. These data convinced Congress that liver transplant was the "preferred treatment for end-stage liver disease" and in 1984, liver transplantation's designation was officially changed to a therapeutic service.[23]

Starzl calls this period "the liver transplant goldrush of 1984."[24] Tilney identifies this as the beginning of the "industrial phase" in transplantation because it entailed an increase in the number of institutions offering transplantation as well as the realization that immunosuppression had the potential to become a big business. No longer a fringe interest of bold surgeons, transplantation had become "a commercially sponsored or underwritten area of medicine,"[25] and part of a movement toward an "increasingly research-directed, technology-based and pharmaceutically oriented thrust of medicine."[26] As such, it's been a huge success. Liver transplantation is now offered as a treatment option for pretty much all causes of liver failure – hepatitis B and C, alcoholic liver disease, non-alcoholic steatohepatitis, cancer, autoimmune liver diseases, metabolic disorders, and acute liver failure from toxins like Tylenol.

Tilney expresses ambivalence about the "industrial phase" of transplantation and its aftermath. On the one hand, he espouses the view that the growth of transplantation is wonderful, but he simultaneously acknowledges that it is complicated. In medicine, surgeon and author Atul Gawande argues that we have a shared belief that medicine is "winning" against illness and mortality,[27] a mindset that medicine is advancing and correspondingly, that "humanity is gaining." But it is not always clear that we are winning. The growth of transplantation has entailed "an escalation of technological commitments."[28] The demand for transplants can only be met through enormous amounts of knowledge, technology, and resources, and an ongoing search for solutions that will require more even knowledge, technology, and resources: better drugs for patients, more viable organ donors, and high-tech solutions like genetically-modified xenotransplants (modifying animal organs to work in humans) and bioengineered synthetic organs. Tilney's bittersweet conclusion is that the success of transplantation has, in fact, created "more arcane, less solvable problems."[29]

A stormy winter evening about ten years after Shauna died, I accidentally gave my two-year-old daughter, who had come down with a fever, too much Tylenol. It was a stupid mistake and I panicked. On the drive to the children's hospital, I concluded that I had caused acute liver failure and therefore my daughter would need a transplant. The nurse tried to turn us away at triage, completely unconcerned because the Tylenol dosage I gave to my daughter was under the daily limit for her size and weight. She nonchalantly advised me not to give her any more Tylenol until the morning, as if *more* Tylenol were even under consideration.

The nurse expected me to leave the hospital and go home, maybe after apologizing for this injudicious visit to the Emergency Department. But I felt stunned and paralyzed. Though I don't recall what I actually did or said, my odd behaviour made her send us back to the waiting room. Not long afterwards, someone brought us into a consultation room and, cutting to the chase, asked me rather gravely: "Is there something you're not telling us?" I collected myself enough to convince this person that I was not withholding. I admitted that I had overreacted, and then we went home.

The answer to that question ("Is there something you're not telling us") was a clear "Yes," but I didn't know where to begin. The Tylenol incident was not actually a close call. My daughter remembered it as the time I gave her too much "medicinecation" and was more upset that we lost her mitten somewhere on the way to or from the hospital. For me, it had triggered fear that on the surface seemed related to potentially endangering her life (even though my daughter was fine) but was actually generated from a deep-seated feeling that everything could go wrong, related to my experience with Shauna.

As time has passed, it seems increasingly absurd to me that the reality of dying on the waitlist remained unspoken. There was no discussion of the kind of death waiting for a transplant may lead to, so I was dramatically unprepared for my sister's death. As far as I can tell, nothing has changed in this regard in the last twenty years. Information on how to prepare for a transplant and what to expect during recovery was readily available. However the possibility of being delisted, or of death, was not explored.

A close friend who knew I had unprocessed feelings about Shauna's death suggested that I read psychologist Francis Weller's writing about grief. He critiques the way we avoid dealing with loss by turning it into something saccharine and redemptive. Weller argues that instead, we should encounter grief and embrace it. By giving grief our attention, we can turn it into something vital and potent that will energize us (what he calls "the wild edge of sorrow").[30] I was not giving grief my attention. Something was subtly erased every time I acknowledged Shauna's death by saying she "died waiting." It's not a neutral description. To "die waiting" smuggles in a hopeful outlook and an orientation to a happy ending.

Moreover, saying Shauna "died waiting" was interlocked with the many taboos around death that we actively kept in place (and are kept in place by the culture of biomedicine and transplantation). Shauna was privately thinking about her mortality, and I am left with only little inklings of this. For instance, I see that on one occasion she wrote in her journal: "Who are the people who die waiting?" The question itself implies the people who die are invisible, unknown entities. It also suggests that she was secretly thinking: will it be me?

Renee Fox and Judith Swazey note that organ transplantation is not oriented to the "medical commons" (or helping more people meet basic healthcare needs) as much as the survival of fortunate individuals and their personal success.[31] While there is talk about transplantation being a technological development for the greater good, the stakes and drama of transplantation are tied to the survival of individual patients. This observation is borne out by my personal experience. For me, the idea of survival was competitive; indeed, the dictionary defines it as "the act or fact of living or continuing longer than another person or thing." Shauna's liver transplant was all about survival. I saw liver transplantation as the only thing that would save her from dying. This reason, and this reason alone, is why I thought liver transplantation was a good thing.

The history of organ transplantation has always foregrounded the impact of individual success stories. In the early days of kidney transplantation, the most notable success story was that of the Herrick twins. In December 1954, Dr Joseph Murray at Brigham Hospital in Boston transplanted a kidney, donated from Ronald Herrick, into Richard, his identical twin. Richard "unexpectedly rapid[ly] transform[ed]" from "a terminally ill individual to one who had completely recovered." Strikingly, Richard even returned to "normal life," married, and had children with one of the nurses who had cared for him in the hospital.[32] The other standout case was John Riteris, who, in 1959, went on to have a "normal life" after receiving a kidney graft from his non-identical twin. Tilney states that Riteris "became in principle the single most important case, psychologically and otherwise, in the history of the field of clinical transplantation."[33] He even claims Riteris's survival was "more influential" than the fact that the majority of transplant patients died.

A narrow focus on individual success stories also shaped the way policy about organ transplantation evolved. A prime example is the congressional hearings on liver transplantation in 1983 to determine whether liver transplantation was "experimental" or "therapeutic." There was very little clinical data available at the time to make that determination. The success of liver transplantation was represented by only twenty-eight individuals who had survived twelve months post-surgery. According to policy scholar Richard Rettig, Thomas Starzl, spearheading the campaign, chose a successful strategy to persuade Congress: personal testimony from the patients themselves, or in the case of pediatric patients, from their parents.[34] The message centred on the individual plight of patients and the benefit of liver transplant in their lives.

These congressional hearings garnered media attention. Rettig highlights an excerpt from ABC's *Nightline* that aired on 14 April 1983. Host Ted Koppel asks guest Thomas Starzl to explain why liver transplant is "not experimental." Starzl responds that there are patients who have successfully received a transplant and resumed their normal lives. Koppel tells him he is "begging the question" because, he points out, there are failures also. He asks, "What if we turn to the failures?" Starzl answers: "I think the fact that there are failures is probably irrelevant because there are failures in any form of therapy. What one looks at is that there can be stunning success and in significant numbers."[35]

Starzl's position that failures are not worth considering is striking. He is saying that if transplant is beneficial to even a few, it justifies our not thinking about the experience of others for whom it fails. This point of view runs through his memoir. Despite drawing attention to the "silent mortality" of transplantation (a phrase Starzl uses several times in his memoir), he heroizes the patients who survive. In his words, "Failure was abundant but success was spectacular."[36] He ends his memoir with a tribute to the "heroic" patients who, through will and courage, represent the "glory of striving." The survivors are the ones who have the "remarkable stories." For surgeons like Starzl they are the "rewards" of the demands and sacrifices they have made in their careers.

Starzl's dismissal of Koppel's suggestion to "turn to the failures" is revealing of a wider context. Namely, patient stories that support the paradigm of progress (recovery, survivorhood) are validated by the institutional, political, and ideological conditions of organ transplantation, and by Western biomedicine and society more broadly. It's all part of the same framework. As anthropologists Lock and Nguyen argue, "Biomedical technologies are not autonomous entities: their development and implementation are enmeshed with medical, social and political interests that have practical and moral consequences." An investment in the notion of human progress binds them together, namely the idea that the development of science and technology will result in the "advancement of humankind."[37]

We are obsessed with progress and improvement. Anthropologist Anna Lowenhaupt Tsing writes that "categories and assumptions of improvement are with us everywhere. We imagine their objects every day: democracy, growth, science, hope." Progress, she argues, has a strong grip on our imagination and thinking outside of progress is an "imaginative challenge." In fact, she writes, "*Progress still controls us even in tales of ruination.*"[38]

Lowenhaupt Tsing's arguments come from her book *The Mushroom at the End of the World*, a fascinating ethnography of wild mushroom hunters in the Pacific Northwest of the United States. The mushroom hunters she writes about experience conditions of precarity and "life without the promise of stability." She argues that these kinds of stories are typically ignored (even though they are "endemic to globalized capitalism") because "progress stories have blinded us" and orient us to a dream version of modernization, a fantasy of living in a "controlled world" where endless improvement is possible. As she puts it, we march to the "driving beat" of progress. But accordingly, this forward-looking tendency means that we don't "notice other temporal patterns" and we "ignore and neglect what doesn't fit the timeline of progress."[39]

Lowenhaupt Tsing argues that we over-rely on the lens of progress, assuming that "the trope of progress is sufficient to know the world." It determines how we understand both *success and failure*. She writes, "The story of decline offers no leftovers, no excess, nothing that escapes progress."[40] Failure is understood only in its relationship to progress rather than inspiring us to examine how failure can be another story entirely. The story of failure in organ transplantation hasn't been adequately told because it hasn't been adequately acknowledged. Failures creep in only as a sense of ambivalence or ghostliness. Tilney, for example, acknowledges that "heart-breaking tragedies" and sad experiences may result in "professional ambivalence." And for all his praise of the exalted lifesaving capacity of transplantation, Starzl acknowledges that "ghosts remain."

Bud Shaw, one of Starzl's liver transplant fellows, wrote a candid memoir, *Last Night in the OR*, that describes a surgical career haunted by ambivalence.[41] Starzl doesn't get an entirely flattering treatment in the book, being described as "acting like a god in the operating room," admonishing the rest of the team, and repeating a mantra about "life" ("I don't want anyone here who doesn't believe in life!") that makes him sound like a zealot. Indeed, Shaw found Starzl so difficult to work with that during one surgery, he was tempted to punch him in the side of the head.[42]

Nonetheless, Shaw was attracted to the heroics and machismo of performing transplant surgery. The sense of control was enthralling to him; it was particularly the thrill of defeating death that made him feel most powerful. He explains, "I felt a kind of wildness that wasn't so much victory as escape, thrilling escape from near death [any patient could die during surgery]. I was a beast and I daily walked up to the brink and jumped in, ripping and tearing and slashing and screaming, always crawling out the other side reaping air and worshipping the weight of my bones." Shaw offers vivid descriptions of the surgeries themselves and the harrowing attempts to stop patients from bleeding to death. His descriptions accentuate the volume of blood involved, pooling in his shoes and dripping off his balls. The stress (and often sleep deprivation) induced a high (or a mania): "Living on the front lines, trying to save everyone while death seemed so close by, not in the shadows, but right there in those brightly lit rooms where we worked."[43]

Last Night in the OR ends with a childhood memory of a family vacation in Florida. Shaw got a fishhook caught in his foot. His general surgeon father employed a technique he had perfected in his small-town practice to remove the hook quickly and painlessly. Later that day, Shaw recalls, *and this is the last line in the book*: "I pressed my cut foot into the solid edge of the pool and felt the release of a sharp pain shooting through the sole." This unexpectedly poignant line made me think about what the release of buried pain alluded to.

There are obvious themes of loss in the book: Shaw's mother's battle with cancer and her eventual death, his own failed marriage. But loss also reverberates in his relationships with his transplant patients. Notably, Shaw felt uncomfortable when patients treated him like a hero, writing that they "made me panic with all their talk of miracles and saving their lives." He thought of the patients who died, either on the operating table or afterwards, including some of the "successful" cases who did well initially. Now retired, Shaw says that when someone asks him what he misses about transplant surgery, he "struggles to give an honest answer." His scripted response is to say he misses the rewards, the highs, the successes, the camaraderie and teamwork. This gets a "knowing nod." But he writes, "If I begin to remember how rarely things went so well. I usually stop then. These seem to be the answers they expect to hear, so that's enough. If I go on, I lose them. But it's not the whole story, nor the most important part of it, at least for me."[44]

In an essay promoting his book, titled "Real Surgeons Can't Cry: How Writing Healed a Doctor," Shaw admits to the difficult emotions that he tried to shield himself from during his career. These emotions only came to the surface when he started writing. He wonders whether he even would have continued his career in transplant surgery if he had been more "reflective" at that time. He also admits that his colleagues have doubted whether the public would like this questioning perspective, suggesting that they wouldn't be able to understand it.[45] Why probe (pressing the foot on the edge of the pool) only to discover that something that is meant to be painless actually aches? If people only want to hear the hopeful stories that give attention to the rewards of organ donation and transplantation, only successful transplants will get acknowledgment and approval. But the whole story ("turning to the failures") deserves a "knowing nod" too.

I never truly confronted the reality of the diseases Shauna had. Nor did I consider the range of possible transplant outcomes, including surgical complications, rejection, the side-effects of immunosuppression, and perhaps even death. It was like only one story existed: the one in which

Shauna would survive post-transplant. I didn't imagine other versions of this story. The history of transplantation established that it is success that should be heralded, and loss, failure, and death should be hidden. The heroes are the survivors. Life post-transplant should be "normal."

Recently, I read anthropologist Loren Eiseley's book of autobiographical essays called *The Unexpected Universe*. Eisely describes walking along the beach after a storm. He observes the shell collectors going about their business, as well as one lone man rescuing the sea stars he thinks still stand a chance of survival if he flings them back into the ocean before the collectors snatch them. Eisely, on the other hand, just ponders the post-storm carnage. The focus of his contemplation is the creatures who didn't make it. He writes, "I love ... the things beaten in the strangling surf, the bird, singing, which flies and falls and is never seen again ... I love the lost ones and the failures of the world."[46]

Woodlawn Cemetery

Shauna's funeral planning began first thing the morning after she died. The funeral home director gently barraged us with logistical questions about what they should do with the body that was now in their care. So, out of obligation, we made decisions quickly. The funeral would be in a week's time, but without a casket or a body. We didn't want Shauna to be embalmed, looking stiff and waxy, and opted to cremate her the following day.

We had a small impromptu gathering at the funeral home right before she was cremated. We chose not to have Shauna dressed in her nicest clothes. She hadn't worn civilian clothes for months, let alone formal attire, and it seemed too odd and unfamiliar to picture her that way, too dissonant with the Shauna who died. Clothes would have implied continuity between her life and her death, not rupture. The hospital gown wasn't a decent option, so we decided to have her wrapped in a white cotton sheet. The simplicity was striking and suggested a mythical or spiritual state of being.

The funeral home ambience was generic and drab, dominated by bland tones, glossy wood, and artificial plants. After the gathering started, I had the idea to fill the casket with rose petals. Close friends rushed off to the florist to buy dozens of multi-coloured roses and together we tore rose petals from the stems and scattered them around her body. This spontaneity brought creative energy and made the makeshift ceremony feel like the least repressive and numbing experience in months. I want to say the effect was sublime. It left an indelible mark: the configuration of Shauna in the casket, the white sheet, the petals – all on the cusp of immolation.

In contrast, the funeral a week later was miserable. I wanted to give a eulogy but couldn't write one, instead just reading from her journals through tears. I understand that a funeral can be a celebration of life, but in this instance, it really wasn't. It was just too sad. Guests sat sombrely. There were no trappings of celebration aside from champagne, which I drank quite a bit of. Like at any funeral, there was lots of hugging, but this was hardly the tribute my sister deserved. It was still sinking in that what had happened to her was irrevocable; we were no longer waiting for something to change.

In the following days, I was mostly bedridden. There were tasks to do – the sorting and packing of her things, choosing what I would like to keep, engaging in the violation of privacy that comes after someone dies: things done without conscious recollection. For Christmas a couple of weeks later, my parents and I decided to visit Katy and her family at their beach house in North Carolina. We went to the local Episcopalian Church for Christmas Eve mass, but at the service I felt sick to my stomach and called Katy's brother to come take me home so I could go back to bed. The only other thing I remember is going to a hardware store to buy a fire pit to put on the deck. Katy and I liked the idea of sitting outside around a fire during the chilly nights. It didn't happen, though. Katy's dad thought the fire pit was a hazard, so we went back to the hardware store and returned it.

On New Year's Eve, I went out for dinner at a Thai restaurant with a small group of friends in Montreal. Too tired and subdued for festivities, I took a taxi home early. The driver asked about my year, so I told him that my sister had recently died. He was truly sorry. We went on to talk about the Indian Ocean tsunami a few days earlier and lamented the staggering death toll and the scale of the tragedy. The cab driver added, "And your sister was forgotten just like that."

I was still in mourning, it hadn't even been a month, so his tactless words stung. It was insensitive to suggest that the memory of my sister had been wiped out. But he had also voiced an uncomfortable truth – the insignificance of any single human life. For me personally, Shauna's death was the *worst* thing that ever happened. However, in the grand scheme of things, a single death doesn't have significance beyond intimate meanings and personal pain.

That frigid winter in Montreal, I re-enrolled in graduate school and resumed the courses I had dropped in the fall. I had maybe been home a week when I got a call that my ninety-four-year-old grandmother in Edmonton was dying. I rushed straight from the airport to the nursing home, arriving almost as she was taking her last breath. I just had time to touch her face and whisper, "Grandma, it's Anita." I think she heard me say it.

Grandma was staying at the provincial motherhouse of the Grey Nuns and being cared for by the sisters who lived there. This was arranged by her niece, who had a decades-long career at the Grey Nuns' Hospital, starting out as a nurse and climbing up into administrative and governance roles. The atmosphere there was serene and otherworldly, and the place was impeccably clean. While we were waiting for the funeral home, there was a summons to the evening mass. I decided to go because Grandma, a devout Catholic, would have wanted me to. I joined a flock of elderly nuns in their grey garb on their way to the chapel. One sister seemed quite perplexed by the presence of someone from outside their hermetic world. She gazed at my face and asked, "Who are you?" I explained why I was there but for my own self, I had no idea how to answer the question.

Grandma's death meant that I unexpectedly found myself back at my childhood home in Saskatoon, where the funeral would be held. It also demolished the structure of the family; it felt as though the nucleus was ruptured, and not only temporarily; it had been permanently dissolved. It was a change marked by swiftness, the way Grandma was quickly buried in the white snow because no one could bear the January cold.

My mother wasn't at Grandma's funeral. She had stayed in Durham, meticulously organizing Shauna's things, holding on to what she could, and unable to face the death of her mother-in-law so soon after Shauna's passing. My cousin Shannon wasn't there either. She had just gone back to England where she lived with her husband and daughter, having just been in North America for Shauna's funeral. Without Shauna, my grandmother, my mother, and Shannon, I felt unanchored. I had previously imagined that when Grandma died, Shauna, Shannon, and I would spend time together going through Grandma's china, her extensive collection of costume jewelry, her clothes and hats, selecting keepsakes and mementos and assuring some kind of continuity of the family matriarchy. In the end, it was just me, a lone person. I took all the costume jewelry but a year later it was stolen when my apartment was robbed. It didn't feel bad; it felt like being showered with numbness.

The theft of Grandma's jewelry exemplified what Elizabeth Bishop's poem "One Art"[1] expresses about the practice of habituating oneself to loss. I have done this throughout my life with my stolen computers, a vanished hard drive, my book of poems, all my CDs, my sister's pearl ring, a special necklace, all the things forgotten, misplaced, left behind, or accidentally deleted. Of course, we are all surrounded by loss, but as Bishop reiterates in her poem, loss (from small to significant) is not a "disaster."

Bishop's life was filled with tragic losses not mentioned in the poem. She lost both her father (to death) and her mother (to an asylum) when she was a baby, and later, a lover to suicide. I didn't know this about Bishop when I first read the poem. Afterward, what started getting to me was the *guile* of the poem, the guile in even the title: "One Art." The mastery of loss – letting go and acceptance – occurs because it *has* to. You really have no choice so what appears as acceptance may also be a bit of a ruse, or a run-around.

For my own part, I reconfigured and rebuilt my life in a hurried way to avoid lingering on what had happened. I didn't have a breakdown; I steadied myself. Carrying on seemed like the only way to prove to Shauna that I was okay. I imagined she had almost an omniscient awareness of what I was doing such that I believed I was fulfilling her expectations and deliberately becoming more like her. At the same time that I applauded myself for marching forward, I felt deeply passive, as though my life was simply unfolding. As a coping strategy, I aligned myself with the idea that there must be a "grand design" – that everything was happening as it was meant to be, even if it felt all wrong.

For the tenth anniversary of Shauna's death, close friends and family planned a reunion in May in Ocracoke,

North Carolina, a tiny island off the Outer Banks. Though I was greatly looking forward to it, once there I retreated inward, going to bed early each night while others stayed up late on the screened-in porch. Though I couldn't connect with the others, I did feel strongly that there was something inherently cathartic about the ocean. It induces an intense longing that seems to come from the sea itself – a vast expanse of generalized heartache, human troubles, fatality, and loss. Standing on the ocean's shore makes death, loneliness, and separation seem part of normal reality, just the way things are. The ocean has a way of making loss and grief generalizable without reducing its potency.

One of the most painful things for me to admit is that maintaining my bond with Shauna has been harder than I expected. I seldom find significant ways to acknowledge her absence and meaningful ways to memorialize her. For example, I liked the idea of establishing a ritual of burning rose petals on the anniversary of Shauna's death to symbolize her cremation, but fresh rose petals don't ignite easily and they don't incinerate completely. They burn down a little, and only with the help of butane. For the first anniversary of Shauna's death I went to Mount Royal Park in Montreal and started a small illegal fire in the woods with my rose petals and almost an entire bottle of lighter fluid. Another year, I lit a fire in a kitchen pot on the balcony. Neither event evoked much sentiment, certainly not as much as I had hoped it would.

A death anniversary is meant to be a recognition but ultimately it feels like a minimization, as though it were possible that any single date, however significant, would be the time to feel one's loss most acutely. The anniversary of Shauna's death doesn't miraculously conjure sadness and longing, and if I *can* summon those feelings, they often come with anxiety and a sense of guilt and failure. As grief loses rawness it loses focus, becoming scattered throughout different aspects of daily life and other relationships, puncturing little voids.

I have a vintage brown leather suitcase full of a few things that remind me of Shauna – the unfinished cross-stitches, a nearly empty bottle of the lotion she used in the hospital, a portion of her ashes in the keepsake urn (around three tablespoons) along with its pink velvet heart-shaped carrying case with her death certificate tucked in, two framed pictures of Shauna and two pictures of me and Shauna when we were girls, lots of scarves, two boxes of dried rose petals from Shauna's funeral, a few scented candles – Mediterranean fig, ylang-ylang, marine moss, cedar, bergamot, and tobacco – surrounded by lots of packing paper. Some of these things are quite random and seem most poignant to me now because they have spent twenty years in a suitcase.

Mostly, I used up Shauna's things rather than preserve them. I still use her small makeup bag and her Coach wallet. Both are looking battered and shabby. She would be appalled if she knew there are clothes of hers that I still wear – socks for instance, T-shirts that I use as pajamas, black seamless underwear made out of some kind of indestructible synthetic fabric, a turtleneck sweater. More precious than these mundane possessions are the cards, letters, and photographs that I have stored in boxes in my front closet. Because of my messy habits, these boxes have accumulated other documents, paper trails of my life history in unedited bits and pieces that distinctly lack the scaffolding of a narrative. To quote Ciara Kierans, "this [the absence of a narrative] is what loneliness is."[2]

To soothe my ongoing sadness, I have turned to repeat listening of a song about a cowboy mourning his runaway horse, "The Ballad of the Absent Mare," from Leonard Cohen's 1979 album, *Recent Songs*. On top of Cohen's distinctly raw and forlorn voice that is well suited to mourning (like the deep abrasive voice of Patti Smith), the lyrics express nuances of grief and mourning that are familiar to me – disaster, collapse, panic, time moving on, a sense of disorder.

A cowboy grieving a horse has become a heartrending metaphor to me, pointing to something above and beyond the meaning of human relationships. To lose a horse is to lose a strong bond and a sense of unison with another creature. I have learned this by adding "horse" rather than "sister" to my internet searches on "grief" and "loss." Folks talk about attachment to horses with passion, and the human-equine bond is characterized by mutual trust, respect, connection, interest, enthusiasm, energy, attention, cooperation, curiosity, caring, and inspiration. Everything that defined my sisterly relationship with Shauna.

Historian and literary theorist Hayden White notes that metaphors and other figures of speech connect concepts that are otherwise "thought not to be related." They are what he calls "swerves in locution" that show us different ways of expressing ideas, new possibilities for thought, and cast familiar things in new light.[3] Literary scholar Eric Cheyfitz explains metaphor as deriving from our ability "to sustain the simultaneous perception of likeness and difference."[4] Metaphors are particularly useful with experiences that are difficult to grasp or come to terms with psychologically. Sometimes we need a metaphoric renaming in order to create an association that makes our feelings easier to comprehend. I found this to be true by turning to accounts of losing horses as a way of understanding what I felt, losing a sister.

From the time that we were little, Shauna and I were very close. She was a bossy older sister but I happily followed along with anything she asked of me because in my mind, she was the most important person in the world. Dressing up was our favourite game. We had a large blue wooden box for our dress-up clothes – old dresses, scarves, shoes, hats, purses, and jewelry – that served to costume a cast of witches, heroines, and hobos in our made-up stories. We played typical make-believe games but tended to foreground misery, like pretending to be orphans or indigents obliged to eke out a living and fend for ourselves in poverty and hardship. We also had a modest collection of Barbie dolls. We sacrificed one of the Barbies to be the villain who we distinguished by cutting off her hair and dressing her in the dowdy homemade doll clothes sewn by our mother.

I was in awe of Shauna going off to kindergarten one year ahead of me. Kindergarten felt entirely out of my league. I was much more comfortable in the sheltered care of our stay-at-home mom. I was timid by nature, but Shauna wasn't. When she was around four years old, she had her picture in the *Edmonton Journal*; it was a close-up of her face as she shook the hand of an alderman during a children's event at the public library. Shauna is wearing a paper hat with a bow tied under her chin. The hat had something to do with Klondike Days, the big annual exhibition that commemorated the regional history associated with the nineteenth-century Gold Rush. I was there too, probably in one of those hats, but clinging to our mother because I was afraid of crowds and dependent on her for a feeling of safety.

As a child, Shauna had a propensity for piecing things together. She was sharp, perceptive, and equipped to navigate new realms with ease. I was not adept at such things. She eavesdropped on adult conversation while I always tuned it out, and she grasped things about the world that I couldn't begin to comprehend. For example, when we watched *Gone with the Wind* as a family when it aired on television over the course of several evenings, Shauna grappled with the heavy themes of civil war and slavery, finding them disturbing and unsettling. But the movie did not penetrate my thick encasement of childhood oblivion. To my mind, it had no connection to the real world, which for me only consisted of my inner confabulations and everyday experiences.

Shauna's concept of reality was more expansive, and she could reconfigure it according to new ideas and information. Sooner than most other children, especially me, she was beginning to see that the world we live in was structured by history and politics. The older she got, the more curious she became about politics, global events, and social and environmental problems. She honed her acuity for such things on the high school debate team. She took it upon herself to be informed, to the extent that she could in the pre-internet early 1990s. A file cabinet in her bedroom had folders with newspaper clippings related to issues of the day: the destruction of the rainforest, nuclear disarmament, the Meech Lake Accord, women's rights, and the hole in the ozone layer.

Until Shauna got sick, we shared a bedroom. It had twin beds with matching sheets and yellow comforters, metal bed frames plated in a fake shiny brass, and a yellow plastic dome-shaped lamp on the dresser. When Shauna no longer wanted to share a bedroom with me, the extra bedroom in our three-bedroom house (used until then as the piano room) became mine. I decorated my new room in pink and white. I even wanted a canopy bed, the gold star of frilliness, but for my parents that was out of the question. Still, though I had my own quarters, a typically tasteless girlhood bedroom, I didn't really want it. This new boundary between me and Shauna made us separate entities in a way that I had never thought of before. It was a big change.

Shauna was diagnosed with autoimmune hepatitis when she was eleven years old. By that time she had lost weight, and her eyes and skin were yellow-tinged and without any lustre, evidence that hepatitis had been present for a while and that probable cirrhosis was occurring. Once autoimmune hepatitis is set in motion there is no cure. Her treatment consisted of corticosteroids (usually prednisone) and immunosuppressants (azathioprine). It was the side-effect of the prednisone that was the most dramatic, especially when prescribed as a megadose, like Shauna's prescription. It causes water retention, fat redistribution, and increased appetite which leads to weight gain and a distinct phenomenon known as "moonface," or what we called a puffy face. It completely altered Shauna's appearance. The dose of prednisone was eventually tapered down, but the long-term use had another side effect that was revealed over time – growth suppression. Shauna's height stayed at four feet and eleven inches, what she measured at eleven years old.

The two of us, who had once looked so similar, were now radically different. In photos from our childhood, Shauna and I are often wearing matching outfits with tidily braided hair. We looked so similar as sisters that we could sometimes pass for identical twins. The differences between us were miniscule – her eyes were bluer; her blond hair slightly darker and redder. Our cookie-cutter proportions, shapes, and sizes ended with her growth suppression and weight gain, and me growing up tall and slim. The effect on our body images was merciless, a combination of resentment, disdain, guilt, and loathing. My body represented an injustice and betrayal to my sister. Comparisons were unavoidable and the conclusion was inevitable – how much easier it was to be me.

Soon after her diagnosis, Shauna was referred to see a specialist at the Children's Hospital in Calgary. We drove there as a family and stayed with an old friend of my father who lived in a big house with many children, the youngest of whom were twin girls my age. On the day of Shauna's appointment at the hospital, I was sent to school with the twins. Shy and nervous about fending for myself in a strange school with children I hardly knew, I felt dread. I would rather have gone to the appointment, though I didn't say so. After all, I was the lucky one who didn't need doctors' appointments. In these circumstances, luck came with uncertain feelings, feelings of being insignificant, superfluous, or lacking a distinct place. But it turned out that my day at the Calgary elementary school was fine. Everyone was nice to me, and the twins included me in their play at recess. I relaxed into being anonymous and inconspicuous and caught sight of the freedom to be had by loosening the ties of belonging and becoming distant.

I didn't understand what illness was like for Shauna. I didn't even spend much time visiting Shauna in the hospital when we were kids. There was a prevailing attitude that children didn't really belong in hospitals, witnessing illness and suffering, bringing in germs, being noisy and disruptive. And even when I made brief visits, the unfamiliarity of the institution itself imposed a gulf between us. Shauna was inaccessible and removed while I carried on my life as normal. Similarly at home, Shauna's health problems took place largely in a zone of exclusion. I just saw from across a chasm that they required monitoring and management with regular doctors' appointments and blood tests, scopes, and biopsies. The situation was alienating and impenetrable, so I turned inward and brooded.

Even a cursory glance at research on the experience of siblings of chronically ill children suggests that I exhibited some of the common traits, especially as an adolescent: being anxious, depressed, and withdrawn; demonstrating loss of interest, rebelliousness, and emotional suppression. There were other factors that contributed to my developing these traits, such as a beloved aunt dying of cancer, an uncle dying of suicide – glimpses of big unanswerable questions and overall disillusionment. I was unstimulated and uninspired by everything except the music that I listened to, which was either viscerally appealing to my sadness, or kind of loud, edgy, and dissonant.

As a teenager, I was obsessed with the 1990s David Lynch television series *Twin Peaks*. Shauna and I both loved *Twin Peaks* because it was beyond anything we had seen on television, or anywhere: the aesthetic, the offbeat plot lines, the haunting music. Unlike other TV shows that were popular at the time, it was complex: both dark and uplifting, comedic and deeply stirring, romantic but also violent, sinister, and cryptic. We recorded the show on blank VHS tapes and watched the episodes over and over. We both adored the show's protagonist, Agent Cooper, who was unlike anybody we'd ever encountered, real or fictitious. Twin Peaks made us realize how isolated our lives were from anything or anybody intriguing. We perhaps had inklings of this as little girls visiting our grandparents in Medicine Hat, Alberta, where we were awed by the priest at the Catholic church. When attending weekly mass at home in Saskatoon I would sit quietly on the hard pew and tune out the old mumbling priest, but the Medicine Hat priest was young and had a booming voice with the affectation of a Shakespearean stage actor (not that I had seen any Shakespeare) that made Shauna and me giggly. We thought he was very weird and liked to impersonate him when Mass was over. That priest offered a brief and subtle subversion of our bland childhood.

Philosopher Paul Ricoeur argues that a story is a fusion of past, present, and future. We construct plots to "distend" our minds and grasp everything at once, including our memories and our anticipations of the future. The life stories we tell ourselves are critical to our self-identity, specifically for establishing a sense of coherence. According to Ricoeur, coherence of identity implies sameness, uniqueness, uninterrupted continuity, or "immutable substratum." Those "durable properties of character" are established narratives about ourselves.[5]

In many ways Shauna's character was defined by her chronic liver disease. It made her an anomaly. It was also hard for her to fit in because of her determination to make something of herself. In Saskatoon, mediocrity was the norm. Shauna was called an *over*achiever, a concept that reveals negative associations with striving and being ambitious. She cared about her grades and worked much harder than her average peers. Doing so was associated with a perceived lack of social skills, as though an excess of achievement (outside of sports) was compensation for being, by social standards, a loser. In Shauna's case, the idea of overachievement also suggests a concern that, given her poor health, she was overextending herself, taking on too much. But working hard was a form of distraction from her liver disease and a way to deny her illness. Her accomplishments were a good subterfuge, drawing attention elsewhere. It created the appearance of thriving that she couldn't project if she spent time in bed doing nothing.

I played a part in constructing this narrative that Shauna was thriving. My expectation that she would always be strong, ambitious, and capable despite her illness shaped both how I saw myself and the way our identities were intertwined. I accentuated her "overachievement" by joining the apathetic crowd in high school and developing an identity shaped by early 1990s grunge, the heyday of messy appearances and teenage alienation. Later on, we developed a dynamic of dependency; I relied on her to be my role model and guide as I entered into early adulthood with a skillset vastly less evolved than hers. I admired Shauna for being so much more accomplished than I was, but I also see that I encumbered her with extraordinary expectations to tackle her obstacles, get on with life, and show me how to do it too. I imposed this on her.

Shauna moved to Toronto to go to university while I was stuck in Saskatoon during my last miserable year of high school. Our letter-writing became a lifeline to me. She had been to Toronto once before on a family trip in 1985 when we stayed with friends at a nondescript high-rise in the suburbs and visited tourist attractions like the CN Tower, dining at the revolving restaurant at the top of the tower that offered a 360-degree view of the city. We also dropped in on our mother's friend Sue, who lived in a Victorian house in Cabbagetown, a formerly derelict neighbourhood in downtown Toronto in the throes of gentrification. The house was narrow, with high ceilings, dark wood details, art on the walls, and pink paint in the dining room that cast a warm, pleasant glow. The dimensions of the house and the density of the neighbourhood were unlike anything Shauna and I were familiar with, and we instantly fantasized about living there. It was the cosmopolitan antithesis to the prairie towns we were used to.

Once she moved to Toronto, Shauna had access to better and more specialized doctors. She went to her appointments with a binder in hand to take notes on her lab results, changes to her medications, and any upcoming tests or procedures. She kept her own meticulous medical records and used the internet to research her conditions and become much more knowledgeable. At this point, she and I were communicating directly about her health, unmediated by our parents, and it felt like we were leaving a lot of the unknowns from childhood behind. In those pre-internet days, patients and families had few resources to find disease information, discuss symptom management and treatment plans with other patients, and consider their options. During the early years of Shauna's illness, there had been no one to talk to about these things. Our parents sought a little peer support from the parents of a boy in Saskatoon who also had autoimmune hepatitis. That family decided to pursue holistic non-Western therapies, a decision that seems understandable to me, given that the Western approach to medicine was limited and did not address the underlying causes of autoimmune hepatitis. (It still doesn't.) Treatment could only slow down the development of cirrhosis and the scarring of the liver, staving off liver failure, but the side-effects of treatment, especially prednisone, were not good.

Our parents conformed to the expectations from a previous era in medicine when patients didn't know much and didn't have preferences or opinions. They lacked the communication skills to speak openly with health professionals and ask for clear information. Their tendency was to be silent and unquestioning around doctors. Where Shauna's health was concerned, our parents just took what was told to them and looked for evidence that everything would be fine, even if this was, at best, uneasy hopefulness, or even a form of avoidance.

This does not just apply to how they handled Shauna's illness; it was also evident in other events, like what happened to their baby who died before Shauna and I were born. Our mother never got to hold that baby. After she gave birth, her baby was taken away and pronounced dead. To this day, she regrets that she didn't ask to see and touch the little lifeless body she had nurtured and cherished through pregnancy. Our parents also never requested an explanation for why the baby died. They were told she wasn't strong enough to live, and this was just accepted in sorrow.

Our mother was a secretary, a fate determined early in life by a school administrator who routed her into the vocational stream in high school on the day of her enrolment. Her parents, poor Polish farmers in Southern Alberta, had no particular ambition for my mother and no money to board her at the dormitory, so while she was in high school she earned her keep as a live-in maid for a well-off family in town.

Our mother's family history is harsh and sombre. Her grandfather on her father's side emigrated from Poland to Buffalo, New York, but got sick and died, leaving our great-grandmother destitute in Poland with seven children. Our grandfather, the second-youngest of those children, fought as a soldier in World War I and then emigrated to Alberta in 1928 because of the government plant to develop agriculture on the "unused" land of the prairies. Recruited as an agricultural labourer and offered free passage and board, Grandpa was part of the colonial expansion in western Canada and with it, the erasure of Indigenous sovereignty and land use.[6]

The Great Depression hit soon after Grandpa arrived in Alberta, and nobody knows what he did to survive the first four years he was here. In 1932 he met and married our grandmother, the daughter of Polish immigrants who had come to southern Alberta to homestead in 1906. They started a small farm and lived in a tiny house dimly lit by a kerosene lamp. Our mother was born in 1934. Two baby brothers born after her died of pneumonia. Both of our parents grew up on farms, but our dad's family was better off financially, part of a hardworking, churchgoing settler-colonial (or "pioneer") farming community in rural Saskatchewan.[7] Our father was a Catholic priest when he met our mother. He left the priesthood and married her at Edmonton's City Hall in November of 1972. At the time, she was pregnant with the baby that died on the day that she was born.

Our father's side of the family manifested the farmer's ethic. They embraced working hard, worshipping God, and demonstrating grace, humility, and gratitude for what life has given you. Our father once told me that the most meaningful part of the Bible to him was the Beatitudes in the New Testament, the idea that "the meek shall inherit the earth." But being meek, quiet, unobtrusive, and trusting was also repressive, and led to harbouring regrets and leaving too much unspoken. Silence and stoicism masked secrets and suffering: a family psychology so common that it is a cliché. This also defined the way that Shauna's health problems led to guilt and loneliness for everyone. I felt guilty for being well, while Shauna felt guilty for being sick and the hardship it caused. She once noticed that our parents were reading *Why Bad Things Happen to Good People*, a book about why God allows pain and suffering. In our minds, it cast Shauna's poor health as a form of divine punishment, and we also suspected our parents felt the same way about the death of their first baby. There were never any overt mentions of punishment or indeed, their culpability; these were quiet undertones. Nonetheless Shauna's illness was a constant source of worry that I believe Shauna felt responsible for. As a result, she treated it mostly as a private burden.

In addition to family influences, there's a wider and pervasive cultural expectation to cope with illness as a private burden. We don't see what illness is truly like by framing it, as we often do, as a sign of extraordinary resilience. I bought into the idea that coping with illness just proved how strong Shauna was. I admired her for it. Anthropologist Robert Murphy suspects that putting sick people on a pedestal also relieves the guilt that others may have about being well. I put Shauna on a pedestal without recognizing that it might have burdened her with the task of assuring everyone that illness, however onerous, can be endured, overcome, and ultimately survived.

Shauna's ability to function so highly despite her poor health led me to believe that liver disease and eventually liver transplantation would be integrated into her life with minimal disruption. Sociologist Anthony Giddens argues that "a person's identity is ... to be found ... in the capacity to keep a particular narrative going."[8] The successful transplant narrative was part and parcel of a lineage of stories that constructed Shauna's identity as someone who had the will and fortitude to manage her illness. Oliver Sacks writes, "When things fall apart, when our plans fall apart, it is by reference to storied projections of life and self."[9] The prospect of a transplant was met with already entrenched notions of Shauna-ness that made it seem like it was *nothing* she couldn't handle. Our sense of her identity was embedded in the "successful" transplant story.

When that story fell apart, it felt like an undermining of her identity, an affront to the person that she was.

Ricoeur argues that the loss of a "narrative configuration" can amount to loss of "personal identity," and that the disintegration of narrative can equate the disintegration of identity.[10] That's why Shauna's death felt like such a profound erasure, an offence against an "immutable" aspect of who she was. She physically died, but on another level (the "lacking a narrative" level), she disintegrated.

In the spring of 2005, five months after her death, I went back to Durham for the graduation ceremony at Duke University. The university had decided to award Shauna her PhD posthumously. She hadn't finished her dissertation before she died, but her advisor and some of Shauna's colleagues in the department brought it to completion. The graduation felt like the culmination of the years that Shauna spent absorbed in the competitiveness of the academic scene, vying for awards, scholarships, and other distinctions. While that world was stressful and full of pressure, Shauna was in her element as a graduate student, both socially and academically.

After the ceremony, there was a graduation party. In an odd way, it was like Shauna's life could be celebrated and somehow carry on without her, like she was in a state of limbo where she wasn't fully gone and could still reach new milestones. A chapter of Shauna's dissertation was published in a special issue of *The History of Political Economy* on the theme of public support of the arts (volume 37, number 3, fall 2005). The volume was dedicated to her memory and the editor of the journal wrote, "The history of economics has lost a bright light and a warm colleague."

After graduation, we went to the Outer Banks in North Carolina to scatter some of Shauna's ashes in the Atlantic Ocean. May was typically warm in North Carolina but the day we scattered the ashes was cold. Our friend Katy swam out in a wetsuit to dump a small plastic bag of Shauna's remains while everyone watched her from the windy shore.

Only a few of Shauna's ashes were scattered. On a single occasion, Shauna had made a passing mention that when she died, she would like her ashes to be scattered in the ocean. But my mother couldn't stand the idea of letting her disappear into the sea like she'd never existed. Our family has a burial plot in Saskatoon's Woodlawn Cemetery and, in the end, most of Shauna's ashes were buried there. My parents want to be buried next to Shauna in Saskatoon when they die. They have already prepaid for their interment and even bought their tombstone.

As for me, I've kept a small amount of Shauna's ashes in a tiny keepsake urn. Eventually, I may even dig up Shauna's ashes from the Woodlawn Cemetery and take her to the ocean like she wanted, maybe even to the Bay of Fundy. I am torn about overriding my parents' wishes, but fundamentally I knew Shauna better than anyone else did. We had a depth of understanding that was mostly unspoken, an ineffable sibling bond rooted in the intertwining of our identities, our shared history, and the central drama of Shauna's illness that defined our childhoods. As young adults, we cultivated a desire to escape the past and the way it had stifled us. Both of us left Saskatoon with the conviction of never going back. Removing Shauna's ashes would be a symbolic gesture that restored some integrity to her ruptured story.

The Hepatic Happening

The conventions of the typical transplant narrative are incompatible with Shauna's death, and I can't easily offer another story in its place. I can only look backward to understand how my perspective has changed over time as I have sorted through memories and layers of reflection with some degree of critical detachment. This retrospection doesn't capture what "really happened," but it does reveal how my perspective on Shauna's death has evolved.[1]

Mark Freeman, author of a book called *Hindsight*, writes, "We do not know, and cannot know, where the story in which we are engaged will lead. The result is that there is a perpetual slippage, an existential gap, between immediate experience and its retrospective transformation through narrative. The present, despite its presence, is characterized by a kind of absence ... There is something missing now, in my immediate experience."[2] The open-endedness and uncertainty of experience is resolved only after the fact. Hindsight produces insight into human existence because, as Freeman rightly contends, "We are frequently late in our understanding of things."[3]

In hindsight, I see that I tied so much purpose and meaning to an imaginary happy ending: Shauna's future free from illness. When our lives are defined by such projected scenarios, we commit what literary scholar Stephen Crites calls the "formal error" of "treating [the future] as if it were past." He explains that, in contrast, "the future is vague and sketchy, incomplete and thin," properly "more like a loose scenario" without a certain outcome. When we allow the future to determine the plot structure of our lives, we give a "specious pastness" to the future. Crites explains that "in a well-strung narrative, reinforced by its closure, by apparent completeness of its action ... The specious future ... will appear as necessary as the past." But the future is really more like a "free unchoreographed dance" or "improvisatory harlequinade." Narrative conventions manufacture a future "rendered more finished than the one that the Harlequin can in fact go careening into."[4]

I think Shauna knew that what she was going through had more in common with an "improvisatory harlequinade" than a fairy tale with a happy ending. She referred to her future liver transplant as a "hepatic happening." Hepatic is the medical term for "related to the liver." A "happening" can simply be defined as an "event or an occurrence." It is also an art term coined in the late 1950s meaning "a partially improvised or spontaneous piece of theatrical or other artistic performance, typically involving audience participation." Examples of famous happenings include Allan Kaprow's 1961 work *Yard*, which "involved the random scattering and piling of tires over the floor and an invitation to visitors to climb over them"; Marta Minujin's *Reading the News* (1965), wherein the artist wrapped herself in newspaper and lay down in the river until all the newspaper had slowly dissolved; and Jean Tiguely's self-destructing sculpture *Homage to New York* (1960), "composed of bicycle wheels, motors, a piano, an addressograph, a go-cart, a bathtub, and other cast-off objects" that smouldered and burned to ruins over the course of a thirty-minute performance piece.[5]

Calling it a "hepatic happening" is therefore an ironic way to refer to a liver transplant. According to Hayden White, irony is distinguished by knowingness and the speaker's recognition of the "poorness of the comparison." This is what makes irony the most complex of the figures of speech – it includes "reflection of the inadequacy of the characterization" and adds layers of meaning that are self-critical and self-reflexive.[6] Meaning is not wholly fixed but instead emergent as irony, according to White, "tries to understand itself."[7]

The critical meaning that emerges from calling it a hepatic happening is that it reframes liver transplantation to highlight the thrown-together or contingent aspects of our lives. It has no plot structure; rather it draws attention to the uncertainty that spirals around without guardrails, or the promise of an ending where everything is resolved. Narrative scholars have noted that we "cannot abide the loathsomeness of contingency" so we are drawn to interpret our lives with the narrative logic of causality: events unfolding according to a plot with a beginning, a middle, and an end.[8] However, while plot can organize "the multiple scattered events" of our lives, the plot structure of narrative can misrepresent "the fundamental indeterminacy of life."[9] In grappling with Shauna's death, my brain would always return to the figurative device of the hepatic happening. Even before I started this project, I wrote a poem called "The Hepatic Happening." It made the point that Shauna's transplant was "unscripted from the start." I described waiting as "the unspooling of unplottable materiality" toward "a vagrant ending." I characterized the deterioration of her health as "the capricious improvisations of demise" and "a free-f(or-)all." I ended the poem cryptically:

The Hepatic Happening

No way to describe the rest of the performance
Maybe some saw the coherent shape of a downward spiral;
a definite crash;
Or find nothing;
Hollow out a cave;
Find nothing but darkness in the hollowed-out cave;
Or find the words ydnuf fo yab eth; Circling back upon itself.

"Ydnuf foy ab eth" is the Bay of Fundy in reverse. It goes back to the beginning of the story.

EPILOGUE

The Bay of Fundy

exulanis
n. the tendency to give up trying to talk about an experience because people are unable to relate to it – whether through envy or pity or mere foreignness – which allows it to drift away from the rest of your story, until it feels out of place, almost mythical, wandering restlessly in a fog, no longer even looking for a place to land.
                      John Koenig, *The Dictionary of Obscure Sorrows*[1]

Mark Freeman describes the ending as the "final episode of an emerging pattern, an evolving story, integrally related to what has come before."[2] Looking backwards allows us to read "the end in the beginning and the beginning in the end."[3]

In the summer of 1985, our family embarked on a cross-Canada road trip. This trip was more ambitious than anything we had done previously. The map of my childhood up until that point included only four places: Saskatoon, Edmonton, Yorkton, and Medicine Hat, a prairie universe. Of those four places, Edmonton was the best. It ranked higher than Saskatoon by a landslide. Not only did Edmonton greatly outsize Saskatoon, it was the home of the West Edmonton Mall, a conglomerate of attractions unrivalled by anything else on the Canadian Prairies. In fact, at that time, it was the largest mall in the entire world.

Shauna and I were dazzled by Edmonton, but we didn't have much to compare it to besides Yorkton and Medicine Hat. Yorkton, a city of about 15,000 three hours from Saskatoon, was noteworthy because it was home to Shannon, our much-admired older cousin. Shannon was pretty and had the aura of the alpha female of a junior high. Her aesthetic echoed the pages of YM and *Seventeen*, which to our minds represented the cutting edge of fashion. Shauna and I wore her hand-me-down clothes proudly and tried our best to imitate her. Shannon was the reason we could go to Yorkton, Saskatchewan, and come back feeling like we had just become much cooler. Shauna and I were far less enthusiastic about going to Medicine Hat, Alberta, to visit our maternal grandparents. Grandma spent most of the time sitting in a sunny chair by the back door looking over the garden. She took a mountain of pills every day and wore the thickest glasses I had ever seen. Grandpa drank buttermilk. Their old house felt like it was from a different era – the furniture, the appliances, the small wooden cabinet in the exterior wall for milk delivery. Going to Medicine Hat was like going back to a time when life was dull and there was nothing interesting to do.

That summer of '85, we were very excited to drive from Saskatoon all the way to Newfoundland in our old white Ford LTD. Our mother borrowed a directory of bed and breakfasts from the local public library to choose our accommodations. She had an aversion to motels, and bed and breakfasts were a thrifty choice. They had quaint names like "Old Oak Farm" and "Happy Apple Acres," and their hosts were friendly and informative retired couples eager to share suggestions about their region. Wanting an alternative to standard motel rooms and more local experiences makes a lot of sense to me now, but it certainly didn't to children in the 1980s. The idea of staying in strangers' homes seemed abnormal to me and Shauna. To us, ages eight and ten, they were just old houses, interesting only to old-fashioned people.

One of the final destinations of our trip was the Bay of Fundy in New Brunswick. The size and intensity of the tides at the Bay of Fundy are a so-called wonder of North America. High tide brings in fifty feet of seawater weighing one hundred billion tonnes; and low tide exposes dramatic rock formations that loom high above the ground. During low tide, tourists can descend a staircase to the ocean floor and walk around until the four storeys of seawater return.

At low tide, the Bay of Fundy evokes an uncanny feeling, the power of the ocean *in absentia*. It's like lying down on a train track even if you know that the freight train is miles off, because it is only a matter of time until it returns. The geometry of the bay, its vast size and depth, its funnel shape, and the oscillation of deep waves in the continental shelf rock the sea with much more intensity than the ordinary gravitational pull of the sun and the moon. There are pictures of me and Shauna standing on the muddy ocean floor, rocky arches in the background, looking small and vulnerable. They mark the origin of Shauna's ill-fated medical story.

After we visited the Bay of Fundy Shauna wasn't feeling well and developed a rash on her back and her chest. Our parents were worried enough that they took her to a walk-in medical clinic the next morning. The doctor there thought it was an allergic reaction but Shauna had no known allergies, so our mother found his diagnosis strange. In addition, other than our visit to the Bay of Fundy, there had been nothing out of the ordinary about the previous day.

Shauna was fatigued for the rest of the trip, but the rash eventually faded. I wasn't sleeping well either. On the ferry from Newfoundland I had watched *The Neverending Story*, a movie based on a German fantasy novel that was the most terrifying and sad thing I had ever seen. There was a blood-thirsty pack of yellow-eyed wolves but the real antagonist in the film is a black swirling cloud called the Nothing, a mysterious entity that erases people and places. The lasting impact of the movie was something intangible that I really couldn't cope with. It also seemed to correspond to our mother's trepidation that something had happened at the Bay of Fundy, and her intuition that things were not as they had been before.

Over the course of that year, there was a drop in Shauna's energy. Our parents took her to the family doctor who had an office in a tiny strip mall on the closest busy street to our house. This doctor was elderly and odd. I didn't like him because he had once prescribed pills for my chronic bedwetting when I was only four years old (I have learned since drugs are not often used to control bedwetting). The only pills I had ever taken before were small pink chewable children's aspirin tablets with a pleasant powdery flavour. No one mentioned not to chew my first bed-wetting pill. The acrid taste made me cry inconsolably.

Shauna not only had fatigue but had started showing jaundice in the whites of her eyes when she saw that bizarre quack/family doctor. He was not that concerned about her symptoms, though, and like the doctor in New Brunswick, he thought they indicated allergies. His sketchy diagnosis was that Shauna had an allergy to *yellow flowers* and recommended setting a dish of her pee in the sun to confirm. Somehow our parents found this assessment trustworthy and reasonable. They didn't take her to a different doctor (which they later regretted). Real information only came to light after Shauna suffered a cold and went to a clinic for a chest X-ray. It revealed an enlarged spleen, a potential sign of liver damage. The doctor at the clinic was alarmed by Shauna's symptoms and referred her to a pediatrician at the hospital, who took her on as a patient and ordered blood tests and a liver biopsy.

Having a pediatrician at that time was exceptional. They were scarce in Saskatchewan and tended to deal only with serious and complicated cases, not the primary care of healthy children. Shauna's pediatrician was caring and diligent. After a phone consultation with a doctor at the Hospital for Sick Children in Toronto, he diagnosed Shauna with autoimmune chronic active hepatitis.

Autoimmune hepatitis is a rare disease that is idiopathic, meaning that no one knows what causes it. It is essentially an attack on the liver by one's own immune system, causing inflammation and scarring. This was explained to us as Shauna's immune system being "overactive," mistaking the liver as foreign, as though confused about its own identity. It hardly seemed plausible. The diagnosis wasn't cataclysmic but it was still alarming, like a brush with the unfathomable.

Our mother saw the Bay of Fundy as a trigger for Shauna's illness, but the rest of the family never really took her seriously. The association seemed random, circumstantial, and too dramatic. At the same time, it was also the closest thing to an explanation we had. Autoimmune diseases are mysterious, even incoherent. Unknown causality made Shauna's illness seem like an inner violation; at least blaming the Bay of Fundy could externalize it and map it onto preconceived notions I had that illness and disease were something foreign, not something that originated from within.

It started as a joke to quip that Shauna had the Bay of Fundy disease. She and I thought it was a clever way to amalgamate her autoimmune disorders (with her subsequent diagnoses of inflammatory bowel diseases – Crohn's and colitis – and primary sclerosing cholangitis). The Bay of Fundy entered into our sisterly lexicon as a place that was a source of contamination and impending doom. We taunted each other with dulse – the thick, reddish, and chewy seaweed snack that the bay is known for – and the mineral-rich salt that's harvested there and sold to tourists. Shauna once mailed me a Burt's Bees bath product called a "Detox Dulse Bath" from the "unpolluted waters of the Bay of Fundy." She adorned it with poison signs and wrote on the package, "Dear Anita, I dare you to have this bath!" Now it seems to me that we were mocking the prospect of Shauna's mortality, but it didn't seem that way at the time, when we didn't know how things were going to end.

We never believed that Shauna was going to die. She had (mostly unspoken) plans to write about her illness. Now I've been left to appropriate her story or at least *meld* it with mine. In the twenty years since she died, what she would have thought and what I think have become indistinguishable to me. I've imagined the following conversation:

ME: Do you remember when Ollie [our cat] won a year's supply of cat food?
SHAUNA: Yes, wasn't that a Purina Pet Food Sweepstake? Wasn't it the grand prize?
ME: No, I don't think it was the grand prize. I think the grand prize was money, like ten thousand dollars or

something that would have seemed enormous to me at the time. I remember filling out the entry form, cutting it off the box of Tender Vittles, and sending it in. The year's supply of cat food was like third prize or something.
SHAUNA: Still, I think we were quite shocked that you won.
ME: I know!
SHAUNA: Didn't you just get sent a bunch of vouchers?
ME: Yes. It was like more cat food coupons than you could possibly imagine.
SHAUNA: I don't think you have won anything ever since.
ME: I haven't. Do you think luck is finite?
SHAUNA: No.
ME: Do you think I used up too much luck when I won that cat food sweepstake?
SHAUNA: No.
ME: Maybe I did.
SHAUNA: No.
ME: It would have been lucky for you to have gotten a liver transplant, though. Much luckier than cat food.
SHAUNA: Especially that cheap cat food we fed Ollie.
ME: You never really cared about Ollie. Not the way I did.
SHAUNA: You whined and cried to get that cat. Like it was the end of the world.
ME: I had no perspective.
SHAUNA: You needed that cat as your ally, though. You felt all alone. Isn't that what we learned in family therapy?
ME: Ha. Do you think you are unlucky?
SHAUNA: That's a dumb question.
ME: But you died!
SHAUNA: Is that what you think? That it was bad luck?

ME: What then, God?
SHAUNA: It has more to do with God than with cat food.
ME: Hmmmmmm.
SHAUNA: It's too painful to think about. If it's either God or cat food, I am going to go with God.
(Shauna, you did! I mean so many people said you went into "the loving arms of God.")
ME: Am I supposed to say cat food now?
SHAUNA: Winning that cat food was lucky.
ME: If we could do it all over, I wouldn't enter that contest.
SHAUNA: If we could do it all over, we wouldn't go to the Bay of Fundy.

"We didn't just think it funny; we both felt deep down some tug, some old wish to believe again in something that was close to our hearts."[4]

(Shauna exits. Gone.)

Notes

INTRODUCTION

1 For Canadian data, see Canadian Institute for Health Information, "Summary Statistics on Organ Transplants, Wait-Lists and Donors," https://www.cihi.ca/en/summary-statistics-on-organ-transplants-wait-lists-and-donors. For US data see Organ Procurement and Transplantation Network, https://optn.transplant.hrsa.gov/data.

2 A.J. Kwong et al., "OPTN /SRTR 2019 Annual Data Report: Liver," in "OPTN /SRTR Annual Data Report 2019, special issue *American Journal of Transplantation* 19, no. S2 (February 2021), https://doi.org/10.1111/ajt.16494; Canadian Institute for Health Information, *e-Statistics Report on Transplant, Waiting List and Donor Statistics, 2020* (Ottawa, ON: Canadian Institute for Health Information, 2021), https://www.cihi.ca/en/summary-statistics-on-organ-transplants-wait-lists-and-donors

3 Susan Sontag, "At the Same Time: The Novelist and Moral Reasoning," in *At the Same Time: Essays and Speeches*, ed. Paolo Dilonardo and Anne Jump, 1st ed. (New York: Farrar, Straus, and Giroux, 2007), 219.

4 E.G. Guba and Y.S. Lincoln, "Competing Paradigms in Qualitative Research," in *Handbook of Qualitative Research*, ed. N.K. Denzin and Y.S. Lincoln (Sage, 1994), 114.

5 Sandra Harding, "Strong Objectivity and Socially Situated Knowledges," in *Whose Science? Whose Knowledge? Thinking from Women's Lives* (Ithaca, NY: Cornell University Press, 1991), 138–3; Donna Haraway, "Situated Knowledges: The Science Question in Feminism and the Privilege of Partial Perspective," *Feminist Studies* 14, no. 3 (1998): 577–99, https://doi.org/10.2307/3178066.

6 Ann Jurecic, *Illness as Narrative* (Pittsburgh, PA: University of Pittsburgh Press, 2012), 16.

7 Jeremy T. VanderKnyff, "Framing Death: Politics, Meaning, and the Strategic Communication of Organ Donation Messages in South Carolina" (PhD diss., University of South Carolina, 2015), 119.

8 Lesley Sharp, *Strange Harvest: Organ Transplantation, Denatured Bodies, and the Transformed Self* (Berkeley and Los Angeles: University of California Press, 2006), 109–10.

9 Paul Ricoeur, "Life in Quest of a Narrative," in *On Paul Ricoeur: Narrative and Interpretation*, ed. David Wood (London: Routledge, 1991), 25.

10 Hayden White, "The Value of Narrativity in Representations of Reality," *Critical Inquiry* 7, no. 1 (1980): 24.

11 Rose Richards, "Writing the Othered Self: Autoethnography and the Problem of Objectification in Writing About Illness and Disability," *Qualitative Health Research* 18, no. 12 (2008): 1725, https://doi.org/10.1177/1049732308325866.

LEARNING ABOUT THE ORGAN SHORTAGE

1 David A. Goldberg, Richard Gilroy, and Michael Charlton, "New Organ Allocation Policy in Liver Transplantation in the United States," *Clinical Liver Disease* 8, no. 4 (October 2016): 108, https://doi.org/10.1002/cld.580.

2 Melissa K. Hyde and Katherine M. White, "To Be a Donor or Not to Be? Applying an Extended Theory of Planned

Behaviour to Predict Posthumous Organ Donation
Intentions," *Journal of Applied Social Psychology* 39, no. 4 (2009):
880–900, https://doi.org/10.1111/j.1559-1816.2009.00464.x.

3 M. Pulvirenti, J. McMillan, and S. Lawn, "Empowerment,
Patient Centred Care and Self Management," *Health
Expectations* 17, no. 3 (2014): 309, https://doi.org/10.1111/j.1369-
7625.2011.00757.x. See also A. Bandura, "Self-Efficacy: Toward
a Unifying Theory of Behavior Change," *Psychological Review* 84
(1977): 191–215, https://psycnet.apa.org/doi/10.1037/0033-
295X.84.2.191.

4 The website has since changed its design and copy; I am
describing the version circa 2016.

5 Thomas Hugh Feeley and Shin-Il Moon, "A Meta-Analytic
Review of Communication Campaigns to Promote Organ
Donation," *Communication Reports* 22, no. 2 (2009): 63–73,
https://doi.org/10.1080/08934210903258852.

6 "Facts about Deceased Organ Donation," Canadian Blood
Services, accessed on 24 April 2025, https://www.blood.ca/en/
organs-tissues/deceased-donation/organ-donation-after-death.

7 Arthur L. Caplan, "Beg, Borrow or Steal: The Ethics of Solid
Organ Procurement," in *Organ Substitute Technology*, ed. D.
Mathieu (Boulder, CO: Westview Press, 1988), 61.

8 Nicole Gerrand, "The Notion of Gift-Giving and Organ
Donation," *Bioethics* 8, no. 2 (1994): 135, https://doi.org/
10.1111/j.1467-8519.1994.tb00250.x.

9 R.J. Howard, "Organ Donation: Social Policy, Ethical, and
Legislative Issues," in *Biopsychosocial Perspectives on
Transplantation*, ed. J.R. Rodrigue (Boston, MA: Springer,
2001), https://doi.org/10.1007/978-1-4615-1333-9_3.

10 Jeffrey Prottas, "How Your Attitude Affects Organ
Procurement," *The American Journal of Nursing* 95, no. 8 (1995):
16N–16Q, https://doi.org/10.2307/3471125.

11 For the US, see "Organ Donation and Transplantation
Legislation History," Health Resources and Services

Administration, https://www.organdonor.gov/about-us/legislation-policy/history. For Canada, consult the statutory laws of each province: Alberta Government, *Human Tissue and Organ Donation Act* (2006); British Columbia Government, *Human Tissue Gift Act* (1996); Government of Newfoundland and Labrador, *Human Tissue Act* (1990); Government of Manitoba, *The Human Tissue Gift Act* (1987); New Brunswick Government, *Human Tissue Gift Act* (2004); Government of Nova Scotia, *Human Tissue Act* (1989); Government of Ontario, *Trillium Gift of Life Network Act* (2000); Government of Prince Edward Island, *Human Tissue Donation Act* (1992); Government of Quebec, *Civil Law of 1993 Articles 42, 43, 44* (1993); Government of Saskatchewan, *Human Tissue Gift Act* (1978).

12 Sam D. Shemie et al., "Ethics Guide Recommendations for Organ-Donation-Focused Physicians: Endorsed by the Canadian Medical Association," *Transplantation* 10, no. 5S (2017): S41–7, https://doi.org/10.1097/TP.0000000000001694.

13 Shemie et al., "Ethics Guide Recommendations." See also Margaret Verble and Judy Worth, "The Case Against More Public Education to Promote Organ Donation," *Progress in Transplantation* (December 1996), https://doi.org/10.1177/090591999600600410.

14 See Committee on Increasing Rates of Organ Donation Board on Health Science Policy, *Organ Donation: Opportunities for Action*, ed. James F. Childress and Catharyn T. Liverman (Washington, DC: The National Academic Press, 2006), https://doi.org/10.17226/11643.

15 For insight into the complexities of this issue, see Maeghan Toews and Timothy Caulfield, "Evaluating the 'Family Veto' of Consent for Organ Donation," *Canadian Medical Association Journal* 188, no. 17-18 (2016), E436-E3, https://doi.org/10.1503/cmaj.160752, https://www.cmaj.ca/content/cmaj/188/17-18/E436.full.pdf.

16 Developing a coordinated national public awareness effort was part of the mandate the House of Commons Standing Committee on Health and Health Canada gave to the Canadian Council for Donation and Transplantation in 2002, inherited by Canadian Blood Services in 2008 as part of an overall "system re-redesign." The 2016 "Systems Progress Report from Canadian Blood Services" gives scant attention to reporting on public awareness and education, but describes it as "improved," indicating that "there are many organizations working to increase awareness of organ donation among Canadians. Patient advocacy groups and health charities continue to work diligently to promote the social and economic benefits of organ donation and transplantation." Canadian Blood Services, "Organ Donation and Transplantation in Canada – Systems Progress Report 2006–2015." Available upon request, at OTDT@blood.ca.

DO NOT F--- WITH ME

1 Kirsty Boyd et al., "Living and Dying Well with End-Stage Liver Disease: Time for Palliative Care?" *Hepatology* 55, no. 6 (June 2012), https://doi.org/10.1002/hep.26075. See also Steven P. Wainwright, "Transcending Chronic Liver Disease: A Qualitative Study," *Journal of Clinical Nursing* 6, no. 1 (January 1997): 43–53, https://doi.org/10.1111/j.1365-2702.1997.tb00282.x, and Ida Torunn Bjork and Dagfinn Naden, "Patients' Experiences of Waiting for a Liver Transplantation," *Nursing Inquiry* 15, no. 4 (December 2008): 289–98, http://dx.doi.org/10.1111/j.1440-1800.2008.00418.x.
2 Jill Brown et al., "Waiting for a Liver Transplant," *Qualitative Health Research* 16, no. 1 (February 2006): 119–36, https://doi.org/10.1177/1049732305284011.
3 Judy Lumby, "Liver Transplantation: The Death/Life Paradox," *International Journal of Nursing Practice* 3, no. 4 (December

1997): 231–8, https://doi.org/10.1111/j.1440-172X.1997.tb00107.x. See also Aluko A. Hope and R. Sean Morrison, "Integrating Palliative Care with Chronic Liver Disease Care," *Journal of Palliative Care* 27, no. 1 (Spring 2011): 20–7, PMID: 21510128.

4 Brown et al., "Waiting for a Liver Transplant."
5 M. Susan Baker and Carol L. McWilliam, "How Patients Manage Life and Health While Waiting for a Liver Transplant," *Progress in Transplantation* 13, no. 1 (2003): 47–60, https://doi.org/10.1177/152692480301300110. See also Barbara Kimbell and Scott A. Murray, "What Is the Patient Experience in Advanced Liver Disease? A Scoping Review of the Literature," *BMJ Supportive and Palliative Care* 5 (2015): 471–80, https://doi.org/10.1136/bmjspcare-2012-000435.
6 Jon Johnson and Timothy J. Legg, "Facing an Existential Crisis: What to Know," medicalnewstoday.com, 6 December 2019, https://www.medicalnewstoday.com/articles/327244.
7 Barbara Ehrenreich, "Welcome to Cancerland: A Mammogram Leads to a Cult of Pink Kitsch," *Harper's Magazine*, November 2001, https://harpers.org/archive/2001/11/welcome-to-cancerland/.
8 *Pink Ribbons, Inc.*, dir. Lea Pool, National Film Board of Canada (2011).
9 This is touched on by Lumby, "Liver Transplantation"; Boyd et al., "Living and Dying Well"; Bjork and Naden, "Patients' Experiences of Waiting"; and Brown et al., "Waiting for a Liver Transplant." See also Anne M. Walling and Neil S. Wenger, "Palliative Care and End-Stage Liver Disease," *Clinical Gastroenterology Hepatology* 12, no. 4 (2014): 699–700, https://doi.org/10.1016/j.cgh.2013.11.010; Anne M. Larson and J. Randall Curtis, "Integrating Palliative Care for Liver Transplant Candidates: 'Too Well for Transplant, Too Sick for Life,'" *JAMA* 295, no. 18 (2006): 2168–76, https://doi.org/10.1001/jama.295.18.2168; Benjamin Hudson et al., "The

Incompatibility of Healthcare Services and End-of-Life Needs in Advanced Liver Disease: A Qualitative Interview Study of Patients and Bereaved Carers," *Palliative Medicine* 32, no. 5 (2018): 908–18, https://doi.org/10.1177/0269216318756222.
10   Bjork and Naden, "Patients' Experiences of Waiting."
11   Bjork and Naden, "Patients' Experiences of Waiting." See also Wainwright, "Transcending Chronic Liver Disease"; Brown et al., "Waiting for a Liver Transplant"; Hudson et al., "The Incompatibility of Healthcare Services."
12   Arthur Frank, *The Wounded Storyteller: Body, Illness and Ethics*, 2nd ed. (Chicago, IL: University of Chicago Press, 1995), 32.
13   Robert F. Murphy, *The Body Silent: The Different World of the Disabled* (New York: W.W. Norton, 1987), 20.

DIE WAITING

1   Sharon R. Kaufman, *And a Time to Die: How American Hospitals Shape the End of Life* (New York: Scribner, 2005), 148.
2   Aluko A. Hope and R. Sean Morrison, "Integrating Palliative Care with Chronic Liver Disease Care," *Journal of Palliative Care* 27, no. 1 (Spring 2011), PMID: 21510128.
3   Caroline Sanders et al., "Planning for End-of-Life Care with Lay-Led Chronic Illness Self-Management Training: The Significance of 'Death Awareness' and Biographical Context in Participants' Accounts," *Social Science and Medicine* 66, no. 4 (2008): 990, https://doi.org/10.1016/j.socscimed.2007.11.003.
4   Judy Lumby, "Liver Transplantation: The Death/Life Paradox," *International Journal of Nursing Practice* 3, no. 4 (December 1997): 231–8, https://doi.org/10.1111/j.1440-172X.1997.tb00107.x.
5   A.M. Larson and J. Randall Curtis, "Integrating Palliative Care for Liver Transplant Candidates: 'Too Well for Transplant, Too Sick for Life,'" *JAMA* 295, no. 18 (2006): 2168–76, https://doi.org/10.1001/jama.295.18.2168.

6 The idea that communication from doctors can facilitate "reframing" to allow hope back in comes from David Rieff's memoir of his mother's death: *Swimming in a Sea of Death* (New York: Simon and Schuster, 2008).
7 Vaclav Havel, "An Orientation of the Heart," in *The Impossible Will Take a Little While: Perseverance and Hope in Troubled Times*, ed. Paul Rogat Loeb (New York: Basic Books, 2014), 106.
8 Nancy Ballard et al., "Patients' Recollections of Therapeutic Paralysis in the Intensive Care Unit," *American Journal of Critical Care* 15, no. 1 (2015): 86–94, PMID: 16391318.
9 Margaret Lock, *Twice Dead: Organ Transplantation and the Reinvention of Death* (Berkeley: University of California Press, 2001), 63.
10 Jennie Dear, "What It Feels Like to Die: Science Is Just Beginning to Understand the Experience of Life's End," *The Atlantic*, 9 September 2016, https://www.theatlantic.com/health/archive/2016/09/what-it-feels-like-to-die/499319/.

HIGH QUALITY

1 Margaret Lock, *Twice Dead: Organ Transplantation and the Reinvention of Death* (Berkeley: University of California Press, 2001), 371.
2 Lock, *Twice Dead*, 4.
3 Rebecca Solnit, "The Separating Sickness: How Leprosy Teaches Empathy," *Harper's Magazine*, June 2013, https://harpers.org/archive/2013/06/the-separating-sickness/.
4 Renée C. Fox and Judith P. Swazey, *The Courage to Fail: A Social View of Transplantation and Dialysis* (Chicago, IL: University of Chicago Press, 1974), 28.
5 Renee Fox and Judith Swazey, *Spare Parts: Organ Replacement in American Society* (Oxford: Oxford University Press, 1994), 69.
6 Lock, *Twice Dead*, 206–7.

7   Lock, *Twice Dead*, 196.
8   Jennifer Cindy Lai, Sandy Feng, and John Paul Roberts, "An Examination of Liver Offers to Candidates on the Liver Transplant Wait-List," *Gastroenterology* 143, no. 5 (2012): 1261–5, https://doi.org/10.1053/j.gastro.2012.07.105.
9   Jeffrey Prottas quoted in Fox and Swazey, *Spare Parts*, 69.
10 Lock, *Twice Dead*, 48–9.
11 Lock, *Twice Dead*, 372.
12 Lesley Sharp, *Strange Harvest: Organ Transplantation, Denatured Bodies, and the Transformed Self* (Berkeley and Los Angeles: University of California Press, 2006), 10–14.
13 Sharp, *Strange Harvest*, 15.
14 Sharp, *Strange Harvest*, 83.
15 Lai et al., "An Examination of Liver Offers."

DEATH AT 6:15

1   Pauline Chen, *Final Exam: A Surgeon's Reflections on Mortality* (New York: Vintage, 2007), 148.
2   Atul Gawande, *Being Mortal: Medicine and What Matters in the End* (New York: Doubleday, 2014), 9.
3   Gawande, *Being Mortal*, 7.
4   Gawande, *Being Mortal*.
5   Gawande, *Being Mortal*.
6   Leo Pessini, "Life and Death in the ICU: Ethics on the Razor's Edge," *Revista Bioetica* 24, no. 1 (2016), http://dx.doi.org/10.1590/1983-80422016241106.
7   Pessini, "Life and Death."
8   Margaret Lock, *Twice Dead: Organ Transplantation and the Reinvention of Death* (Berkeley: University of California Press, 2001), 62.
9   Lock, *Twice Dead*, 61–3.
10 In Nicholas Tilney, *Transplant: From Myth to Reality* (New Haven, CT: Yale University Press, 2002), 193.

11 Thomas Starzl, *The Puzzle People* (Pittsburgh, PA: University of Pittsburgh Press, 1992), 165.
12 Ruth Behar, *The Vulnerable Observer: Anthropology that Breaks Your Heart* (Boston, MA: Beacon Press, 1996), 52.
13 Susan Sontag, *Illness as Metaphor* (New York: Farrar, Strauss and Giroux, 1978), 41–2.
14 David Rieff, *Swimming in a Sea of Death: A Son's Memoir* (New York: Simon and Schuster, 2008).
15 Rieff, *Swimming in a Sea*, 42.
16 Rieff, *Swimming in a Sea*, 86.
17 The study was part of SUPPORT (Study to Understand Prognoses and Preferences for Outcomes and Risks of Treatments). See Alfred F. Connors et al., "A Controlled Trial to Improve Care for Critically Ill Hospitalized Patients," *JAMA* 274, no. 20 (1995): 1591–8, https://doi.org/10.1001/jama.1995.03530200027032.
18 Sharon Kaufman, *And a Time to Die: How American Hospitals Shape the End of Life* (New York: Scribner, 2005).
19 Kaufman, *And a Time to Die*, 319.
20 Kaufman, *And a Time to Die*, 323.
21 Kaufman, *And a Time to Die*, 154.
22 Tom Andrews and Alvita Nathaniel, "Awareness of Dying Remains Relevant after Fifty Years," *Grounded Theory Review* 2, no. 1 (2015): 3–10, http://groundedtheoryreview.com/.
23 Robert F. Murphy, *The Body Silent: The Different World of the Disabled* (New York: W.W. Norton, 1987), 64.
24 Lock, *Twice Dead*, 71–2.
25 Kaufman, *And a Time to Die*, 153.
26 Sven Mikulee, "'A Woman Under the Influence': Cassavetes' Intense and Emotionally Exhausting Slice of Life," *Cinephilia Beyond*, n.d., accessed 20 August 2025, https://cinephiliabeyond.org/a-woman-under-the-influence-cassavetes-intense-and-emotionally-exhausting-slice-of-life/.

THE STORY OF MELD

1 Saleh Elwir and John Lake, "Current Status of Liver Allocation in the United States," *Gastroenterology and Hepatology* 12, no. 3 (March 2016): 166–70, https://pmc.ncbi.nlm.nih.gov/articles/PMC4872844/.
2 David A. Goldberg, Richard Gilroy, and Michael Charlton, "New Organ Allocation Policy in Liver Transplantation in the United States," *Clinical Liver Disease* 8, no. 4 (October 2016): 108, https://doi.org/10.1002/cld.580.
3 OPTN data reports are searchable: https://optn.transplant.hrsa.gov/data/view-data-reports/regional-data/.
4 The media attention around Job's transplant made the point that he didn't "cut the line"; see Ray Hainer, "Did Steve Job's Money Buy Him a Faster Transplant?," CNN Health, https://www.cnn.com/2009/HEALTH/06/24/liver.transplant.priority.lists/. I discuss later in this chapter that a cancer patient like Steve Jobs would have had exceptional MELD points (patients with hepatocellular carcinoma are allotted standardized exception points, but Jobs had a rare pancreatic cancer, so his points would have been non-standardized), which may have given him an advantage.
5 Thomas Starzl, *The Puzzle People: Memoirs of a Transplant Surgeon* (Pittsburgh, PA: University of Pittsburgh Press, 1992), 175.
6 Richard Rettig, "The Politics of Organ Transplantation: A Parable of Our Time," *Journal of Health, Policy, Politics and Law* 14, no. 1: 191–227, https://doi.org/10.1215/03616878-14-1-191; see also the Summary of NOTA at https://www.congress.gov/bill/98th-congress/senate-bill/2048?r=5.
7 Richard B. Freeman, "MELD: The Holy Grail of Organ Allocation?," *Journal of Hepatology* 42, no. 1 (January 2005): 16–20, https://doi.org/10.1016/j.jhep.2004.11.002; Eunice Lee, Chris J.C. Johnston, and Gabriel C. Oniscu, "The Trials and

Tribulations of Liver Allocation," *Transplant International* 33, no. 11 (July 2020): 1343–52, https://doi.org/10.1111/tri.13710; Russell Wiesner et al., "Model for End-Stage Liver Disease (MELD) and Allocation of Donor Livers," *Gastroenterology* 124, no. 1 (January 2003): 91–6, https://doi.org/10.1053/gast.2003.50016.

8 Evangelos Cholongitas and Andrew K. Burroughs, "The Evolution in the Prioritization for Liver Transplantation," *Annals of Gastroenterology* 25, no. 1 (2012): 6–13, https://pmc.ncbi.nlm.nih.gov/articles/PMC3959341/.

9 Freeman, "MELD," 17.

10 Nicholas Tilney, *Transplant: From Myth to Reality* (New Haven, CT: Yale University Press, 2002), 262.

11 Freeman, "MELD."

12 Russell Wiesner et al., "Model for End Stage Liver-Disease." See also Patrick S. Kamath et al., "A Model to Predict Survival in Patients with End-Stage Liver Disease," *Hepatology* 33, no. 2 (December 2003): 464–70, https://doi.org/10.1053/jhep.2001.22172. For the Canadian context, see Kelly W. Burak et al., "Validation of the Model of End-Stage Liver Disease for Liver Transplantation Allocation in Alberta: Implications for Future Directions in Canada," *Canadian Journal of Gastroenterology and Hepatology*, 3 April 2016, https://doi.org/10.1155/2016/1329532.

13 Wiesner et al., "Model for End Stage Liver-Disease."

14 Ann Jurecic, *Illness as Narrative* (Pittsburgh, PA: University of Pittsburgh Press, 2012), 22.

15 Jurecic, *Illness as Narrative*.

16 Helen Lambert, "Accounting for EBM: Notions of Evidence in Medicine," *Social Science and Medicine* 62 (2006): 2633–45, https://doi.org/10.1016/j.socscimed.2005.11.023.

17 Iris Marion Young, "Polity and Group Difference: A Critique of the Idea of Universal Citizenship," *Ethics* 99, no. 2 (1989): 250, https://www.jstor.org/stable/2381434.

18 Trisha Greenhalgh et al., "Six 'Biases' against Patients and Carers in Evidence-Based Medicine," *BMC Medicine* 13, no. 200 (2015), https://bmcmedicine.biomedcentral.com/articles/10.1186/s12916-015-0437-x.
19 Greenhalgh et al., "Six 'Biases,'" 2–5.
20 Pauline Chen, *Final Exam: A Surgeon's Reflections on Mortality* (New York: Vintage Books, 2007), 94.
21 Mauro Bernardi, Stefano Gitto, and Maurizio Biselli, "The MELD Score in Patients Awaiting Liver Transplant: Strengths and Weaknesses," *Journal of Hepatology* 54, no. 6 (2011): 1297–1306, https://doi.org/10.1016/j.jhep.2010.11.008.
22 Andres E. Ruf et al., "Addition of Serum Sodium into MELD Score Predicts Waiting List Mortality Better than MELD Alone," *Liver Transplantation* 11, no. 3 (March 2005): 336–43, https://doi.org/10.1002/lt.20329; Shunji Nagai et al., "Effects of Allocating Livers for Transplantation Based on Model for End-Stage Liver Disease – Sodium Scores on Patient Outcomes," *Gastroenterology* 155, no. 5 (November 2018): 1451–62, https://doi.org/10.1053/j.gastro.2018.07.025.
23 "Policy 9: Allocation of Liver, 9.1 A. Adult Status 1A Requirements," in Organ Procurement and Transplantation Network, *OPTN Policies*, effective date 8 January 2025, https://optn.transplant.hrsa.gov/media/eavh5bf3/optn_policies.pdf.
24 Robert J. Fontana, "Acute Liver Failure Including Acetaminophen Overdose," *Medical Clinics of North America* 92, no. 4 (2008): 761–94, https://doi.org/10.1016/j.mcna.2008.03.005.
25 Pratima Sharma et al., "End-Stage Liver Disease Candidates at the Highest Model for End-Stage Disease Scores Have Higher Wait-List Mortality than Status-1A Candidates," *Hepatology* 55, no. 1 (2011): 192–8, https://doi.org/10.1002/hep.24632.
26 Joseph Ahn et al., "End-Stage Liver Disease Patients with MELD > 40 Have Higher Waitlist Mortality Compared to Status

1A Patients," *Hepatology International* 10 (2016): 838–46, https://doi.org/10.1007/s12072-016-9735-4.
27 Freeman, "MELD," 19.
28 David S. Goldberg and Kim M. Olthoff, "Standardizing MELD Exceptions: Current Challenges and Future Directions," *Current Transplantation Reports* 1 (2014): 232–7, https://doi.org/10.1007/s40472-014-0027-4; Saleh Elwir and John Lake, "Current Status of Liver Allocation in the United States," *Gastroenterology and Hepatology* 12, vol. 3 (2016): 166–70, https://pmc.ncbi.nlm.nih.gov/articles/PMC4872844/.
29 Patrick Grant Northup, "Excess Mortality in the Liver Transplant Waiting List: Unintended Policy Consequences and Model for End-Stage Liver Disease (MELD) Inflation," *Hepatology* 61, no. 1 (2015): 285–91, https://doi.org/10.1002/hep.27283.
30 Goldberg and Olthoff, "Standardizing MELD Exceptions," 18.
31 Alina Allen et al., "Reduced Access to Liver Transplantation in Women: Role of Height, MELD Exception Scores and Renal Function Underestimation," *Transplantation* 102, no. 10 (October 2018): 1710–16, https://doi.org/10.1097/tp.0000000000002196; Jayme E. Locke et al., "Quantifying Sex-Based Disparities in Liver Allocation," *JAMA Surgery* 155, no. 7 (May 2020), https://doi.org/10.1001/jamasurg.2020.1129; Monica Sarker et al., "Outcomes in Liver Transplantation: Does Sex Matter?" *Journal of Hepatology* 62, no. 4 (April 2015): 946–55, https://www.ncbi.nlm.nih.gov/pmc/articles/PMC5935797.
32 Omobonike O. Oloruntoba and Cynthia A. Moylan, "Gender-Based Disparities in Access to and Outcomes of Liver Transplantation," *World Journal of Hepatology* 7, no. 3 (2015): 460–7, https://doi.org/10.4254/wjh.v7.i3.460.
33 Jennifer Guy and Marion G. Peters, "Liver Disease in Women: The Influence of Gender on Epidemiology, Natural History,

and Patient Outcomes," *Gastroenterology and Hepatology* 9, no. 19 (2013): 633–9.
34 Locke et al., "Quantifying Sex-Based Disparities."
35 Sarker et al., "Outcomes in Liver Transplantation."
36 C.A. Moylan et al., "Disparities in Liver Transplantation Before and After Introduction of the MELD Score," *JAMA* 300, no. 20 (2008): 2371–8, https://doi.org/10.1001/jama.2008.720.
37 Allen et al., "Reduced Access to Liver Transplantation."
38 Locke et al., "Quantifying Sex-Based Disparities."
39 Jennifer C. Lai et al., "Height Contributes to Gender Difference in Waitlist Mortality Under the MELD-Based Liver Allocation System," *American Journal of Transplantation* 10, no. 12 (2010): 2658–64, https://pubmed.ncbi.nlm.nih.gov/21087414/.
40 Norah A. Terrault et. al., "Liver Transplantation 2023: Status Report, Current and Future Challenges," *Clinical Gastroenterology and Hepatology* 21, no. 8 (July 2023): 2150–66.
41 W. Ray Kim et al., "MELD 3.0: The Model for End-Stage Liver Disease Updated for the Modern Era," *Gastroenterology* 116, no. 6 (December 2021): 1887–95.
42 Wiesner et al., "Model for End-Stage Liver-Disease."
43 Parul Dureja and Michael R. Lacey, "Disparities in Liver Transplantation in the Post-Model-For-End-Stage-Liver-Disease Era: Are We There Yet?" *Hepatology* 50, no. 3 (2009): 981–4.

FAILURE

1 That day he left an envelope with my parents with a note inside that said, "Dear Shauna, it is almost too much to bare [*sic*] that our last meeting on earth has taken place."
2 When Shauna had an organ offer, my father declared in the online journal: "Liberation from disease is dawning."

3   Nicholas Tilney, *Transplant: From Myth to Reality* (New Haven, CT: Yale University Press, 2002), 202–4.
4   Tilney, *Transplant*, 202.
5   Tilney, *Transplant*, 199.
6   Tilney, *Transplant*, 3.
7   Tilney, *Transplant*, 80.
8   Thomas Starzl, *The Puzzle People: Memoirs of a Transplant Surgeon* (Pittsburgh, PA: University of Pittsburgh Press, 1992), 170.
9   Tilney, *Transplant*, 152–3.
10 Barry Kahan, "Organ Donation and Transplantation: A Surgeon's View," in *Organ Transplantation: Meanings and Realities*, ed. Stuart J. Younger, Renee C. Fox, and Laurence J. O'Connell (Madison, WI: University of Wisconsin Press, 1996), 132.
11 Starzl, *The Puzzle People*, 207–8.
12 Tilney, *Transplant*, 173–5.
13 Marina Joubert, "1967: Reflections on the First Human Heart Transplant and Its Impact on Medicine, Media and Society," *Public Understanding of Science* 27, no. 1 (2018): 110–14, https://doi.org/10.1177/0963662517738619.
14 Margaret Lock, *Twice Dead: Organ Transplantation and Reinvention of Death* (Berkeley: University of California Press, 2001), 85. The media attention, however, ultimately contributed to a moratorium of heart transplantation in 1970 as the public became aware of low success rates as well as some questionable practices around organ donation. See Tilney, *Transplant*, 178–9.
15 "CDTRP 10th Anniversary Celebrations – First Edition," The Canadian Donation and Transplantation Research Program website, 25 April 2023, https://cdtrp.ca/en/10th-anniversary-celebrations-first-edition/.
16 Tilney, *Transplant*, 70.
17 Tilney, *Transplant*, 109–10.
18 Tilney, *Transplant*, 96.
19 Tilney, *Transplant*, 113.

20 Tilney, *Transplant*, 117.
21 Tilney, *Transplant*, 129.
22 Tilney, *Transplant*, 232–3.
23 Rettig, "The Politics of Organ Transplantation," 204–5.
24 Starzl, *The Puzzle People*, 257.
25 Tilney, *Transplant*, 254.
26 Tilney, *Transplant*, 281.
27 Atul Gawande, *Being Mortal: Medicine and What Matters in the End* (Toronto: Doubleday, 2014).
28 Harold Moore, "Beyond Survival – Daniel Callahan: The Tyranny of Survival," *The Review of Politics* 37, no. 3 (1975): 418, https://doi.org/10.1017/S0034670500024578.
29 Tilney, *Transplant*, 281.
30 Francis Weller, *The Wild Edge of Sorrow: Rituals of Renewal and the Sacred Work of Grief* (Berkeley, CA: North Atlantic Books, 2015).
31 Renee Fox and Judith Swazey, *Spare Parts: Organ Replacement in American Society* (Toronto: Oxford University Press, 1994).
32 Tilney, *Transplant*, 62
33 Tilney, *Transplant*, 73.
34 Richard Rettig, "The Politics of Organ Transplantation: A Parable of Our Time," *Journal of Health, Policy, Politics and Law* 1, vol. 14 (1989): 199.
35 Rettig, "Politics of Organ Transplantation," 201.
36 Starzl, *The Puzzle People*, 173.
37 Margaret Lock and Vihn-Kim Nguyen, *An Anthropology of Biomedicine* (Oxford: Wiley-Blackwell, 2010), 1–20.
38 Anna Lowenhaupt Tsing, *The Mushroom at the End of the World: On the Possibility of Life in Capitalist Ruins* (Princeton, NJ: Princeton University Press, 2015), 21. Emphasis added.
39 Tsing, *Mushroom at the End of the World*.
40 Tsing, *Mushroom at the End of the World*. Emphasis added.
41 Bud Shaw, *Last Night in the OR: A Transplant Surgeon's Odyssey* (New York: Plume, 2015).

42 Shaw, *Last Night in the* OR, 20–32.
43 Shaw, *Last Night in the* OR, 164–7.
44 Shaw, *Last Night in the* OR, 238–9.
45 Bud Shaw, "Real Surgeons Can't Cry: How Writing Healed a Doctor," *Electric Literature* (15 September 2015), https://electricliterature.com/real-surgeons-cant-cry-how-writing-healed-a-doctor/.
46 Loren Eisely, *The Unexpected Universe* (New York: Harcourt Brace, 1969), 182.

WOODLAWN CEMETERY

1 Elizabeth Bishop, "One Art," https://www.poetryfoundation.org/poems/47536/one-art.
2 "It took me ages to realize that this is what loneliness is; it is the lack of a narrative"; Ciara Kierans, "Narrating Kidney Disease: The Significance of Sensation and Time in the Emplotments of Patient Experience," *Culture, Medicine, Psychiatry* 29 (2005): 34, https://doi.org/10.1007/s11013-005-9171-8.
3 Hayden White, *Tropics of Discourse: Essays in Cultural Criticism* (Baltimore, MD: Johns Hopkins University Press, 1978), 2.
4 Eric Cheyfitz, *The Poetics of Imperialism: Translation and Colonization from the Tempest to Tarzan* (Philadelphia, PA: University of Pennsylvania Press, 1997), 106.
5 Paul Ricoeur, "Narrative Identity," in *On Paul Ricoeur: Narrative and Interpretation*, ed. David Wood (New York: Routledge, 1991), 190–5.
6 For a discussion of agriculture as a tool of colonization see Zoe Matties, "Unsettling Settler Food Movements: Food Sovereignty and Decolonization in Canada," *Cuizine: The Journal of Canadian Food Cultures* 7, no. 2 (2016), https://doi.org/10.7202/1038478ar.
7 As Matties reminds us in "Unsettling Settler Food Movements," the status of "pioneer" negates Indigenous

presence and denies the prior existence and values of Indigenous subsistence activities on the land. The European settler perspective only valued the conversion of land for agricultural use.

8 Anthony Giddens, *Modernity and Self-Identity: Self and Society in the Late Modern Age* (Palo Alto, CA: Stanford University Press, 1991), 54.
9 Quoted in John D. Engel et al., *Narrative in Health Care: Healing Patients, Practitioners, Profession and Community* (New York: Radcliff, 2008), 52.
10 Ricoeur, "Narrative Identity," 196.

THE HEPATIC HAPPENING

1 John A. Robinson and Linda Hawpe argue in their essay "Narrative Thinking as a Heuristic Process" in *Narrative Psychology: The Storied Nature of Human Conduct*, ed. R. Sarbin (New York: Praeger, 1986), 123, that stories change through retrospection and undergo "narrative repair." We "repair" our narratives when after "testing the continued validity of life experience stories" they come up short.
2 Mark Freeman, *Hindsight: The Promise and Peril of Looking Backward* (Oxford: Oxford University Press, 2010), 85.
3 Freeman, *Hindsight*, 26.
4 Stephen Crites, "Storytime: Recollecting the Past and Projecting the Future," in *Narrative Psychology: The Storied Nature of Human Conduct*, ed. Theodore R. Sarbin (Westport, CT: Praeger, 1986), 163-9.
5 "Happenings," *The Art Story*, n.d., accessed 20 August 2025, https://www.theartstory.org/movement/happenings/.
6 Hayden White, *Tropics of Discourse: Essays in Cultural Criticism* (Baltimore, MD: Johns Hopkins University Press, 1978), 5-6.
7 White, *Tropics of Discourse*, 19.
8 Peter Goldie, "Life, Fiction, Narrative," in *Narrative, Emotion, and Insight*, ed. Noël Carroll and John Gibson (University

Park: The Pennsylvania State University Press, 2011). The phrase "loathsomeness of contingency" is a quotation from Frank Kermode, *The Sense of an Ending: Studies in the Theory of Fiction* (Oxford: Oxford University Press, 2000), 147. Kermode is referring to the novel *Nausea* by Jean-Paul Sartre.

9 Ann Jurecic, *Illness as Narrative* (Pittsburgh, PA: University of Pittsburgh Press, 2016), 31–8.

EPILOGUE

1 John Koenig, *The Dictionary of Obscure Sorrows* (New York: Simon & Schuster, 2021), 15.
2 Mark Freeman, *Hindsight: The Promise and Peril of Looking Backward* (Toronto: Oxford University Press, 2010), 41.
3 Mark Freeman, "Data Are Everywhere: Narrative Criticism in the Literature of Experience," in *Narrative Analysis: Studying the Development of Individuals in Society*, ed. Colette Daiute and Cynthia Lightfoot (Sage, 2004), 65.
4 Kazuo Ishiguro, *Never Let Me Go* (New York: Vintage Books, 2005), 67.

Index

autoimmune hepatitis, 123, 128, 142

CaringBridge.org, 8, 37
chemical paralysis, 42, 47, 53
Chen, Pauline, 65, 87

denial, 35–6, 41; of mortality, 65–6, 71; of negative outcomes, 44, 46

Eisely, Loren, 112
end-stage liver disease: patient experience of, 21, 26
evidence-based medicine, 86–7
experience of waiting, 11–12, 24–6, 33–5, 78–9

faith, 43–4, 48–9
family override, 19
fantasy of recovery, 43, 66, 68
Frank, Arthur, 27, 43
Freeman, Mark, 134, 138

Gawande, Atul, 65–7, 72, 103
gift of life, 8, 16, 57, 63–4
good death, 71–2
graft tolerance and immunosuppression, 100–2
grief, 105, 114–15, 117–20

hope, 5, 43–8, 61, 65
hyponatremia, 29–30

ICU experience: invisibility of death in, 71–3; and isolation, 51–4; treatment excess, 66–7
identity, 126–7, 131–3
illness: and battle metaphor, 69–70; concealment of, 27, 126; sibling experience of, 123–5; social expectations and standards for, 26–7, 131
irony, 136

Jurecic, Ann, 6, 86

Index

Kaufman, Sharon, 41, 71–3

life support withdrawal, 73, 75–7
liver failure: ascites, 29, 38; cirrhosis, 29; encephalopathy, 34, 40; spontaneous bacterial peritonitis, 31; symptoms of, 22, 34, 36–41
liver transplantation: history of, 96–7, 102–3, 106–7; limitations of, 95–7; unrealistic expectations for, 46–8
liver transplantation allocation policy: and hepatocellular carcinoma, 90–1; history, 80–2; and status 1A, 88–9
Lock, Margaret, 54, 57–8, 62–3, 67, 72–3, 99–100; and Ngyuyen, 108
Lowenhaupt Tsing, Anna, 108–9

MELD: and disease severity, 92–3; and gender bias, 91–2; and implications of waiting, 82–6; MELD-Na, 88; and mortality risk, 86, 92; and objectivity, 86–7
metaphor, 120
Murphy, Robert, 27, 72, 131

narrative: conventions, 9; hindsight in, 134; plot structure, 126, 136; and reality, 10; and temporality, 135

organ donation: anxiety about, 13; commodification of, 62–4; eligibility for, 15–16, 18–19; and erasure/denial of death, 58, 63; and ethics, 16; and exploitation, 79–80; gap between supply and demand, 7, 11, 17; promotion of, 7–9, 12, 13–15, 20; registration for, 15–17; research, 13–15; tragedies, 56–7
organ offers declined, 58, 60–1
organ transplantation: acknowledgment of failure, 111–12; ambivalence about, 103, 109, 111; history of, 68, 98–9; individual success, 106–7; as liberation, 61, 96; limitations of, 100; public perception of, 99–100

progress: ideology of, 108–9; narratives of, 5, 108

required request, 17–18
Ricoeur, Paul, 9, 126, 132
Rieff, David, 69–70

Sharp, Lesley, 8, 62–3
Shaw, Bud, 109–11
Sontag, Susan, 4, 69–70
Starzl, Thomas, 68–9, 97–9, 102, 107–9

Tilney, Nicholas, 96–7, 99, 101–3, 106, 109

transplant narratives: and happy ending, 6–8, 43, 108; and redemption, 9; and transformation, 8–10

transplant surgery risks, 43, 46

UNOS, 93–4

ventilation, 42, 47, 53

waitlist death: absence of stories about, 4; invisibility of, 104–5; lack of preparation for, 105; statistics about, 3–4, 11, 78

Western biomedicine: discourse, 5; ideology, 6, 65–6

White, Hayden, 10, 120, 136